Mental health refers to a person's emotional, psychological, and social well-being. It encompasses how individuals think, feel, and behave, as well as how they cope with the ups and downs of life, handle stress, and relate to others. Good mental health isn't just the absence of mental illness; it's also about having a positive sense of well-being, feeling capable and productive, and having healthy relationships.

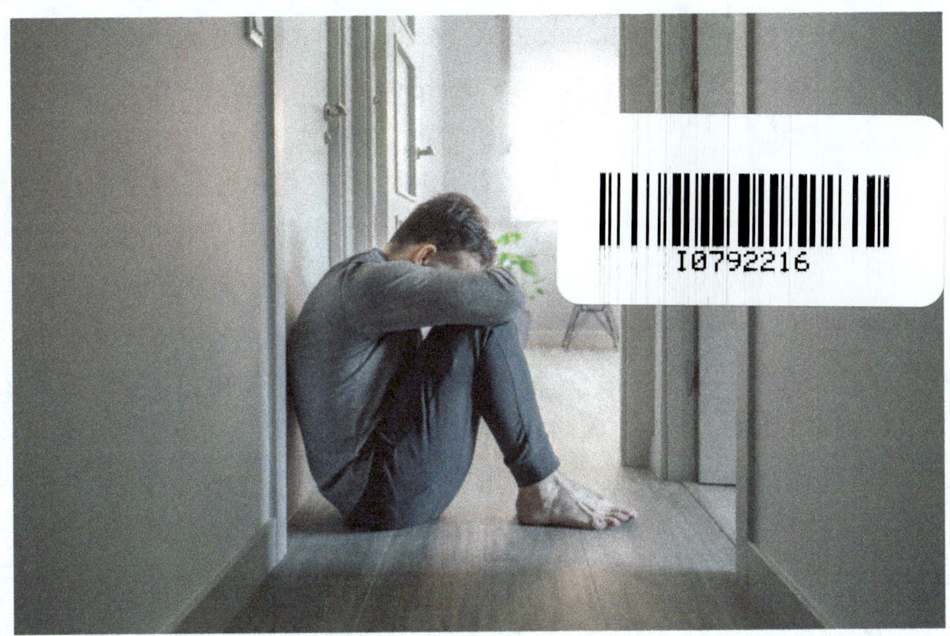

The importance of mental health cannot be overstated, as it significantly influences every aspect of a person's life:

- **Physical Health:** Mental health is interconnected with physical health. Poor mental health can lead to physical health problems such as headaches, digestive issues, and weakened immune system.
- **Emotional Well-being:** Good mental health allows individuals to experience and manage a wide range of emotions in a healthy way. It promotes resilience, enabling people to bounce back from setbacks and cope with stress effectively.
- **Relationships:** Mental health affects how individuals interact with others, form and maintain relationships, and communicate. Strong mental health fosters healthy relationships and social connections.
- **Productivity and Functioning:** When mental health is optimal, individuals can focus, concentrate, and perform effectively at work, school, and in daily activities. It enhances creativity, problem-solving skills, and decision-making abilities.
- **Quality of Life:** Mental health is essential for overall life satisfaction and fulfillment. It contributes to a sense of purpose, meaning, and enjoyment in life.
- **Prevention of Mental Illness:** Prioritizing mental health through self-care practices, stress management, and seeking support when needed can reduce the risk of developing mental illnesses and promote early intervention when symptoms arise.

Understanding Mental Health:
- Overview of mental health and its importance in overall well-being.
- Breaking down the stigma surrounding mental health issues.

Types of Mental Health Problems:

- Anxiety Disorders:
  - Generalized Anxiety Disorder (GAD)
  - Panic Disorder
  - Phobias
  - Obsessive-Compulsive Disorder (OCD)
- Mood Disorders:
  - Depression
  - Bipolar Disorder
- Psychotic Disorders:
  - Schizophrenia
  - Delusional Disorder
- Eating Disorders:
  - Anorexia Nervosa
  - Bulimia Nervosa
  - Binge Eating Disorder
- Substance Use Disorders:
  - Alcoholism
  - Drug Addiction
- Personality Disorders:
  - Borderline Personality Disorder (BPD)
  - Narcissistic Personality Disorder (NPD)
  - Antisocial Personality Disorder (ASPD)

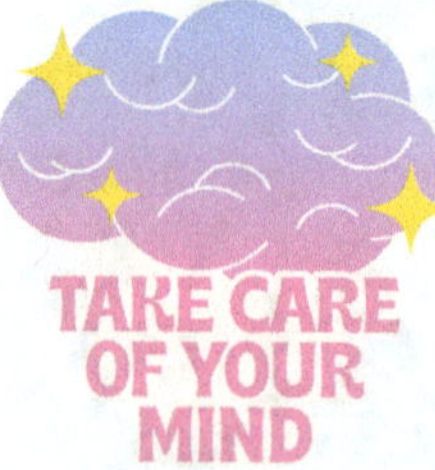

Mental health is not a luxury reserved for a select few; it is a fundamental aspect of human existence that touches us all. Just as we care for our physical health, we must tend to our emotional and psychological well-being with equal diligence. This requires a shift in mindset, away from stigma and shame, towards compassion and understanding.

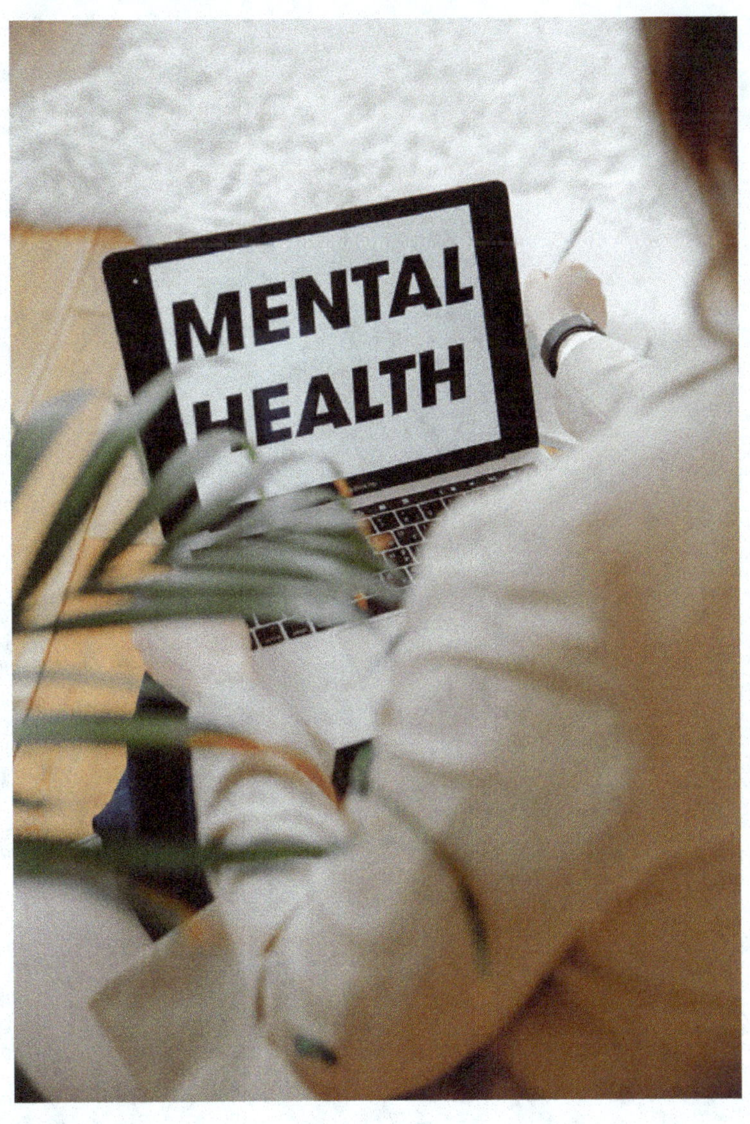

Let us create a society where seeking help for mental health concerns is met with support and encouragement, rather than judgment or silence. Let us foster environments where individuals feel safe to express their emotions, seek assistance when needed, and journey towards healing without fear of discrimination.

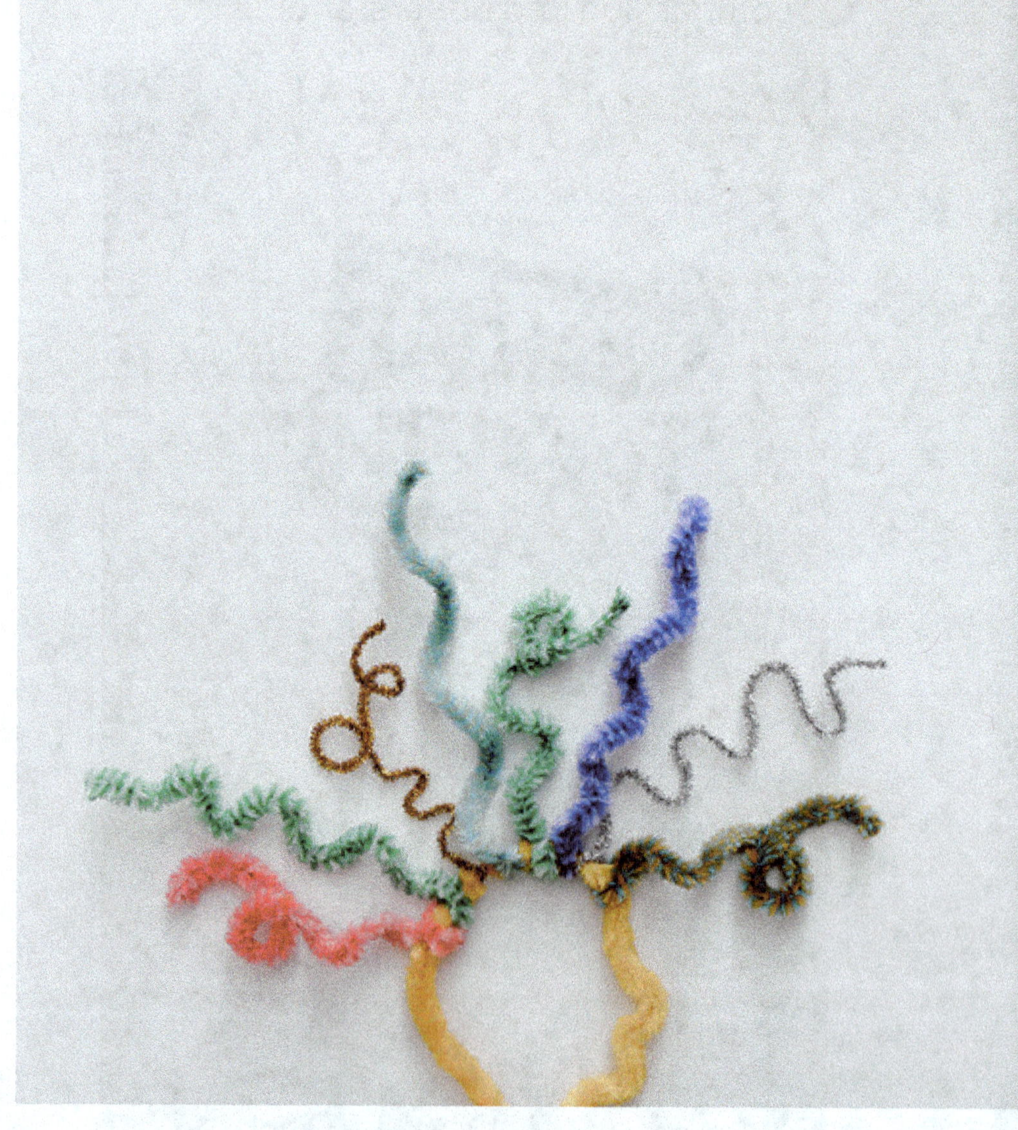

It is within our power, as a society, to dismantle the barriers that stand in the way of mental health access and support. Let us invest in mental health education, destigmatize conversations about mental illness, and prioritize resources for mental health care services. By doing so, we not only uplift individuals in need but also strengthen the fabric of our entire community.

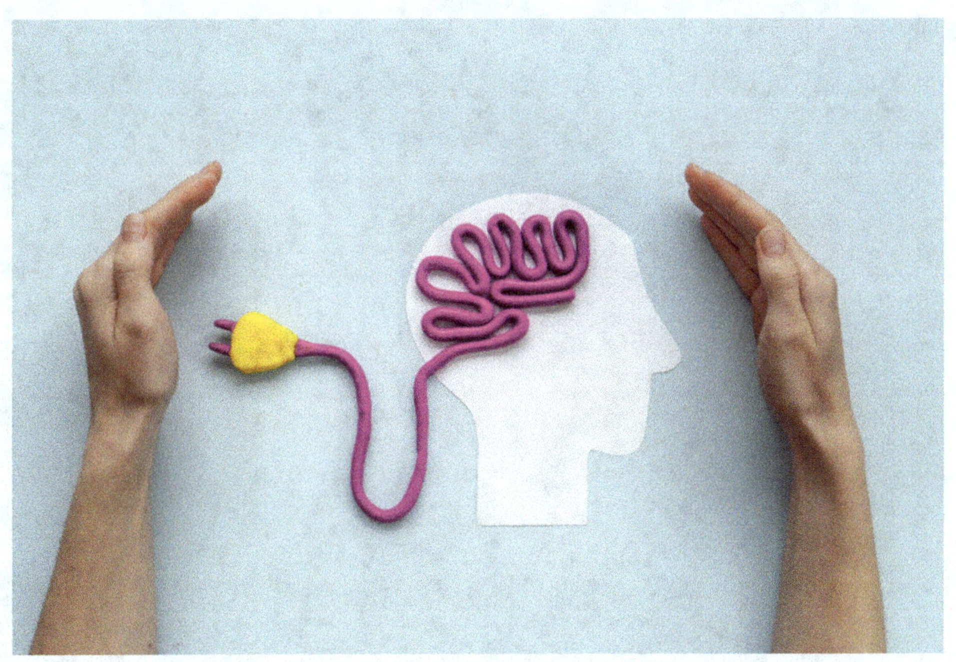

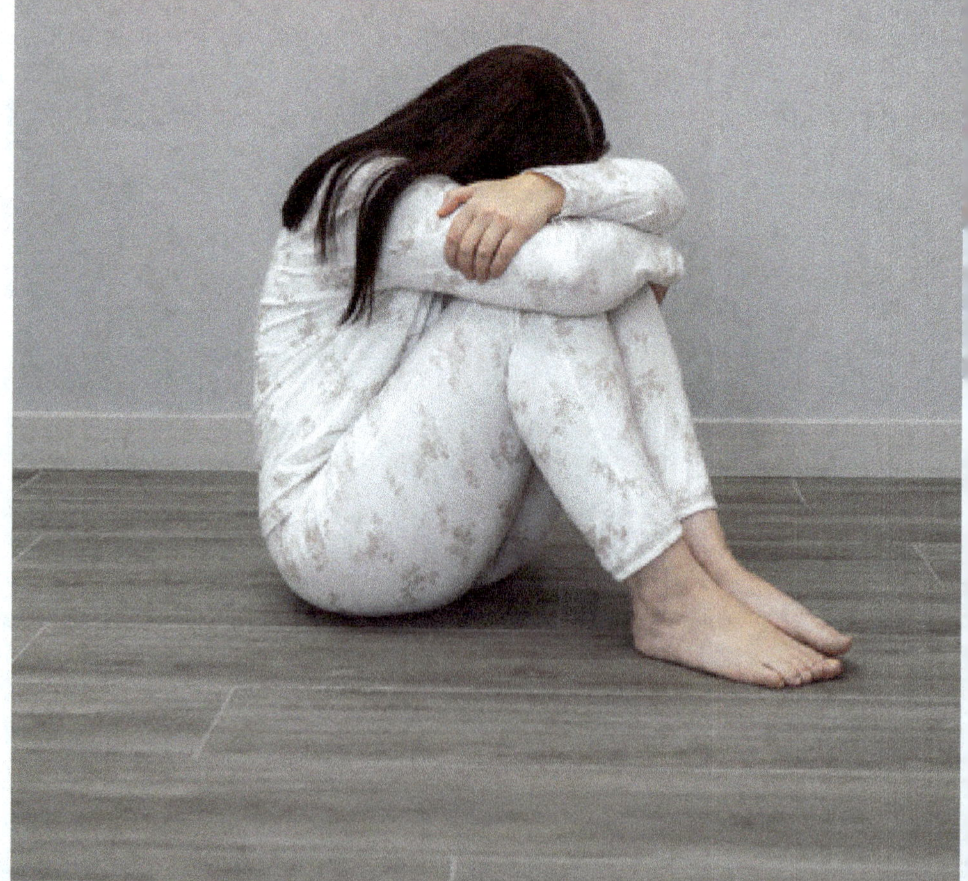

MENTAL
HEALTH
MATTERS

Together, let us build a society where mental health is valued, where compassion is abundant, and where every individual can thrive. Our collective well-being depends on it.

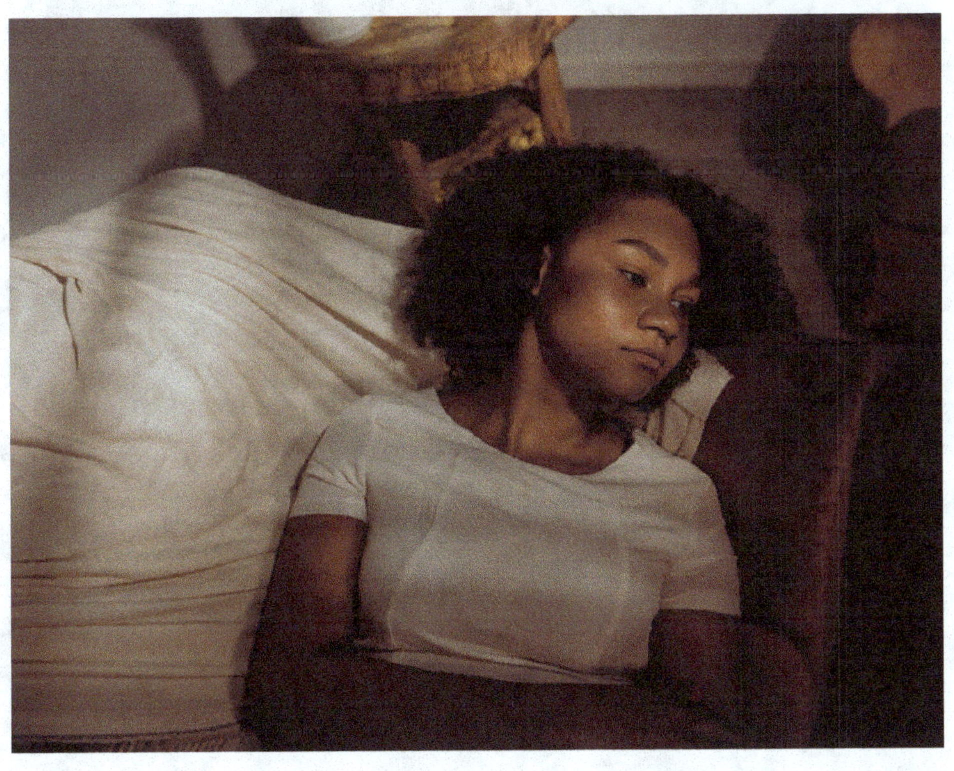

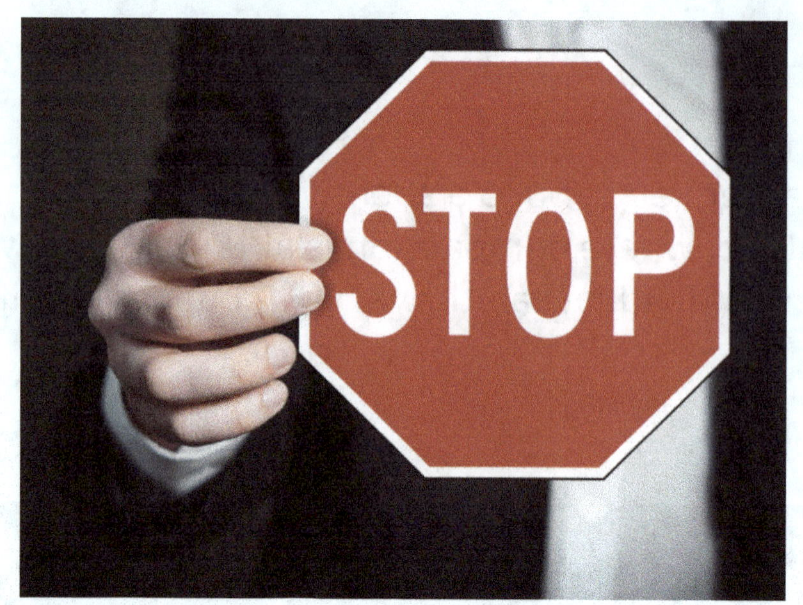

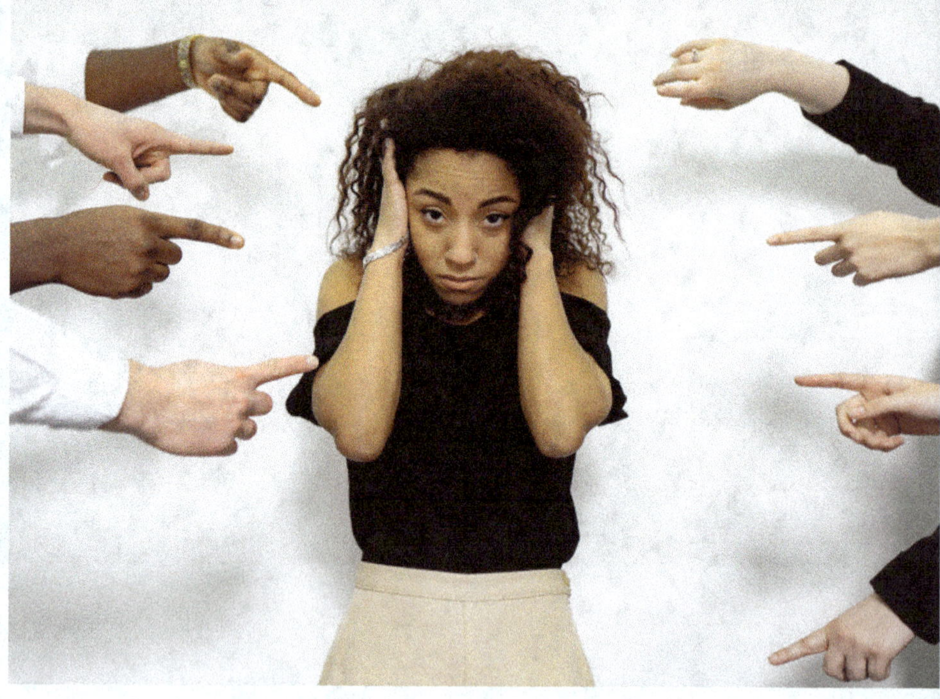

PHYSICAL VS. MENTAL ILLNESS

Physical Illness

Any physical condition that significantly impacts one's daily activities.

Examples

- Flu
- Broken Bone
- Food Allergy

Ways to Address

- Medical Consultation
- Physical therapy
- Medications

Mental Ilness

Any condition affecting emotion, thinking, or behavior and influencing how a person functions.

Examples

- Anxiety
- Depression
- Attention-Deficit/Hyperactivity Disorder (ADHD)

Ways to Address

- Medical Consultation
- Behavior therapy
- Medications

MY SELF-CARE BUCKET

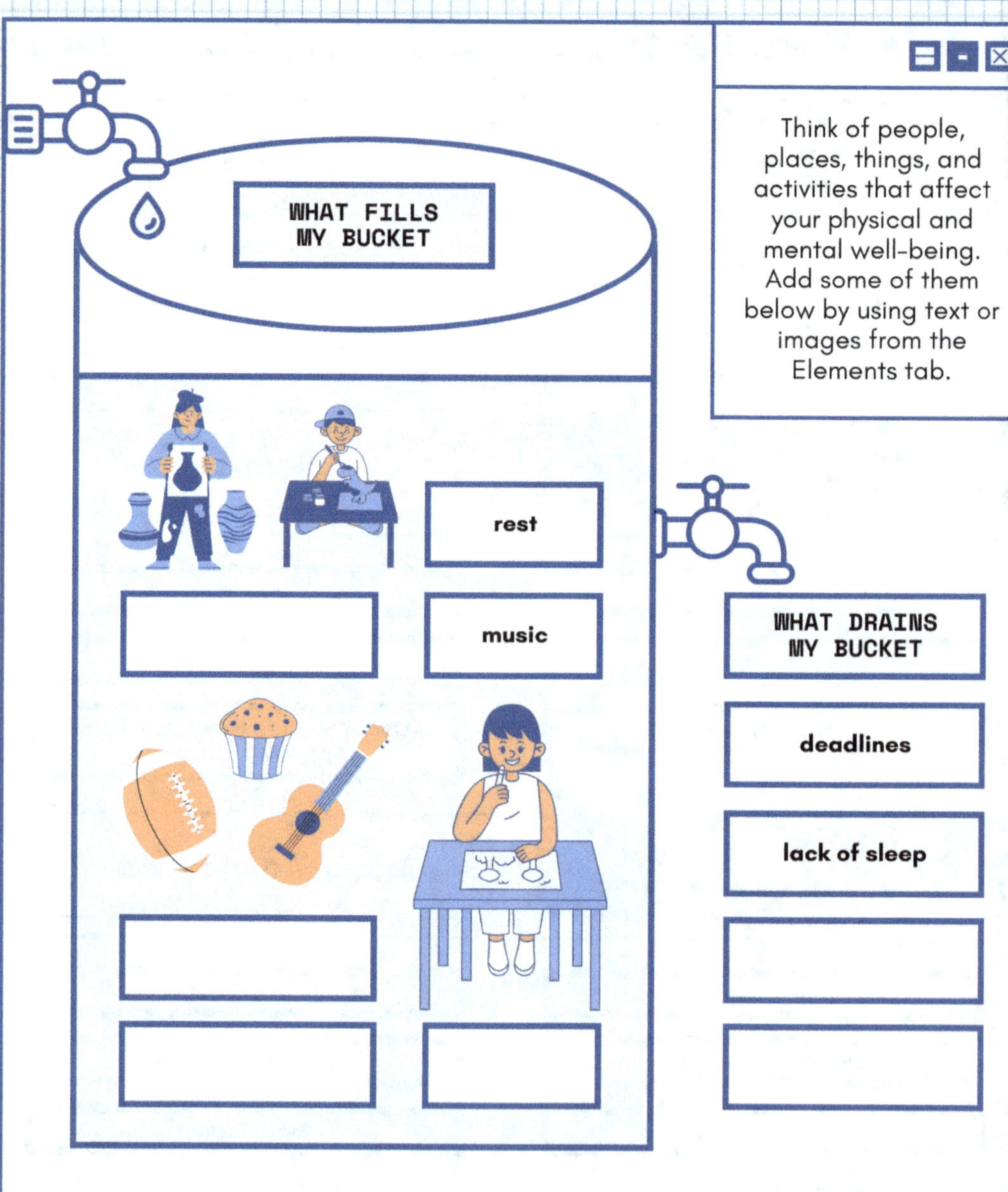

Think of people, places, things, and activities that affect your physical and mental well-being. Add some of them below by using text or images from the Elements tab.

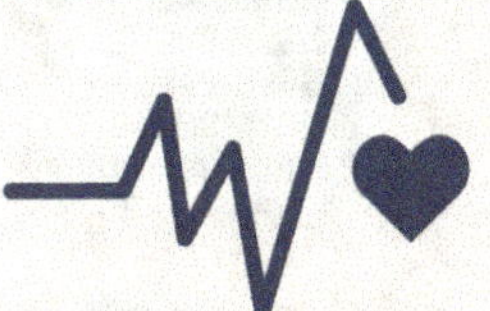

The Importance of Mental

Health Awareness

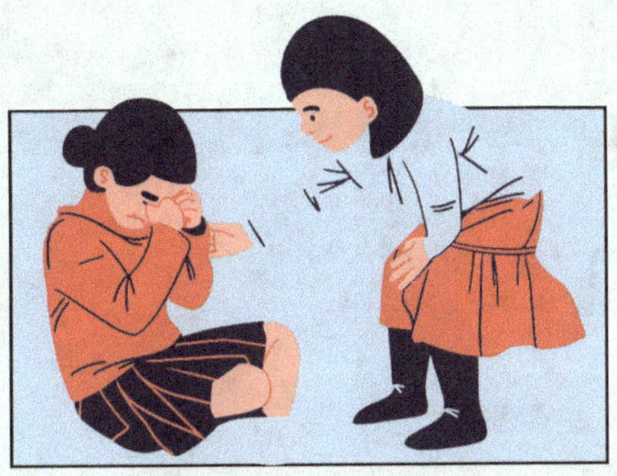

01 Mental health awareness involves understanding and recognizing the importance of mental well-being and the impact of mental health on overall quality of life.

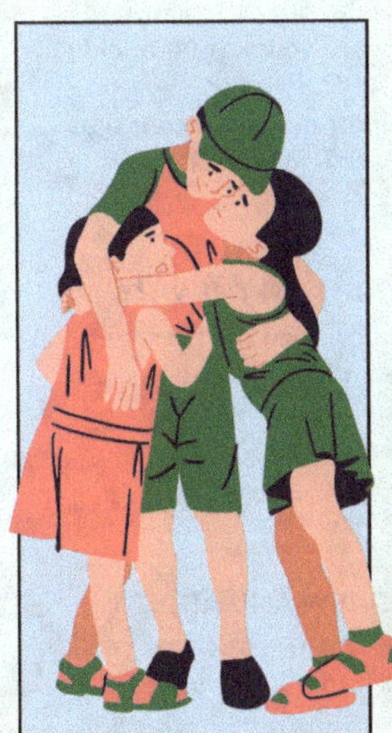

02 Mental health awareness helps reduce stigma, promotes empathy, and encourages open conversations about mental health concerns.

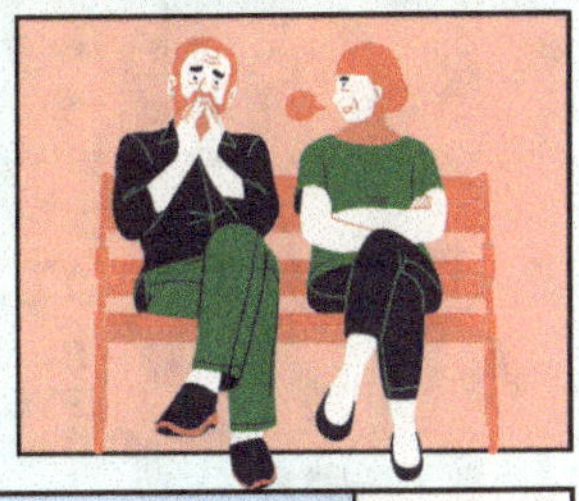

03 Increased mental health awareness leads to early recognition and intervention of mental health issues, improving outcomes and preventing further distress.

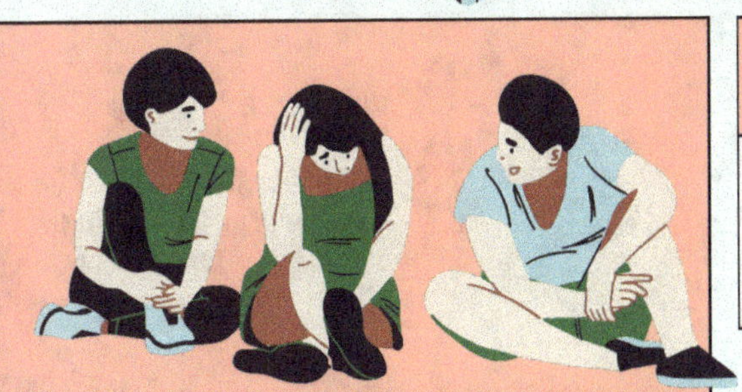

04 Mental health awareness helps reduce stigma, promotes empathy, and encourages open conversations about mental health concerns.

Killer Tips: Develop Effective Habits

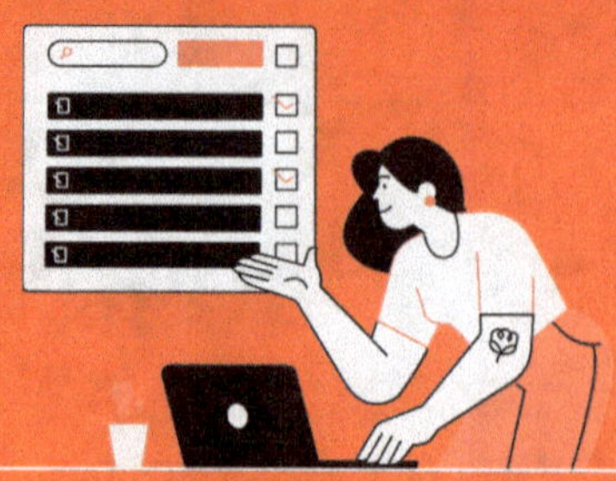

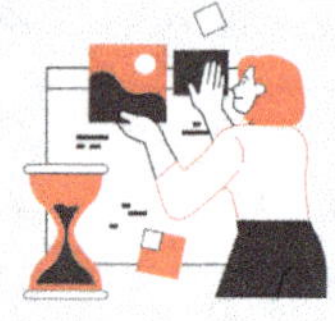

START SMALL AND BE CONSISTENT

Consistency is key, commit to practicing the habit daily to reinforce its development.

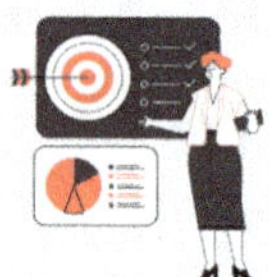

SET CLEAR AND SPECIFIC GOALS

Make your goals measurable, achievable, and relevant to keep yourself motivated.

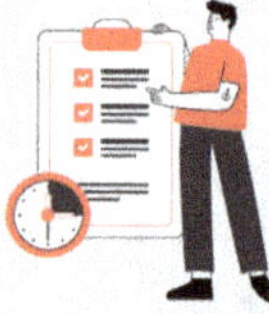

TRACK YOUR PROGRESS

Keep a habit tracker or journal to monitor your daily adherence to the habit.

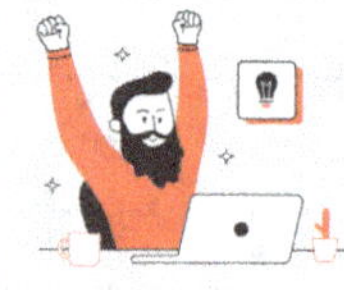

USE POSITIVE REINFORCEMENT

Celebrate small wins and reward yourself for sticking to the habit. Positive reinforcement encourages continued behavior.

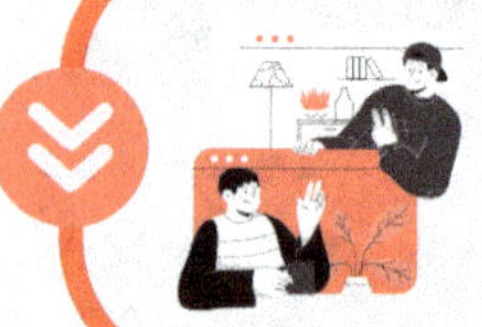

BUILD A SUPPORT SYSTEM

Share your habit-building journey with friends or family who can encourage and support you.

FOCUS ON THE WHY

Understand the reasons behind developing the habit and its positive impact on your life.

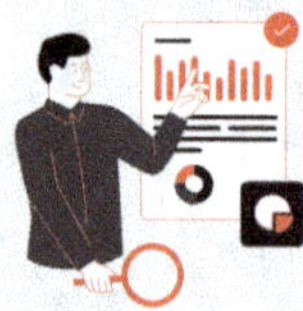

LEARN FROM SETBACKS

Accept that setbacks are a part of the habit-building process. Analyze the reasons for setbacks and use them as opportunities to improve.

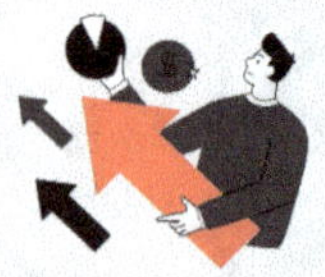

REVIEW AND ADJUST

Visualize yourself performing the habit effortlessly and achieving your goals.

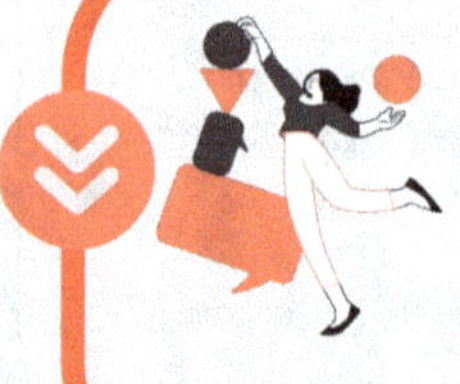

IMPLEMENT HABIT STACKING

Attach the new habit to an existing one that is already well-established. This way, you build on an existing routine to develop new habits seamlessly.

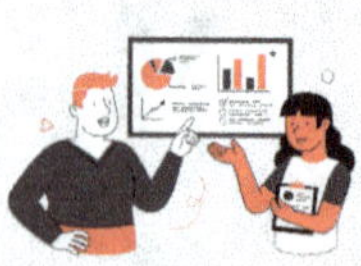

VISUALIZE SUCCESS

Regularly review your habit-building journey and assess the effectiveness of the habit.

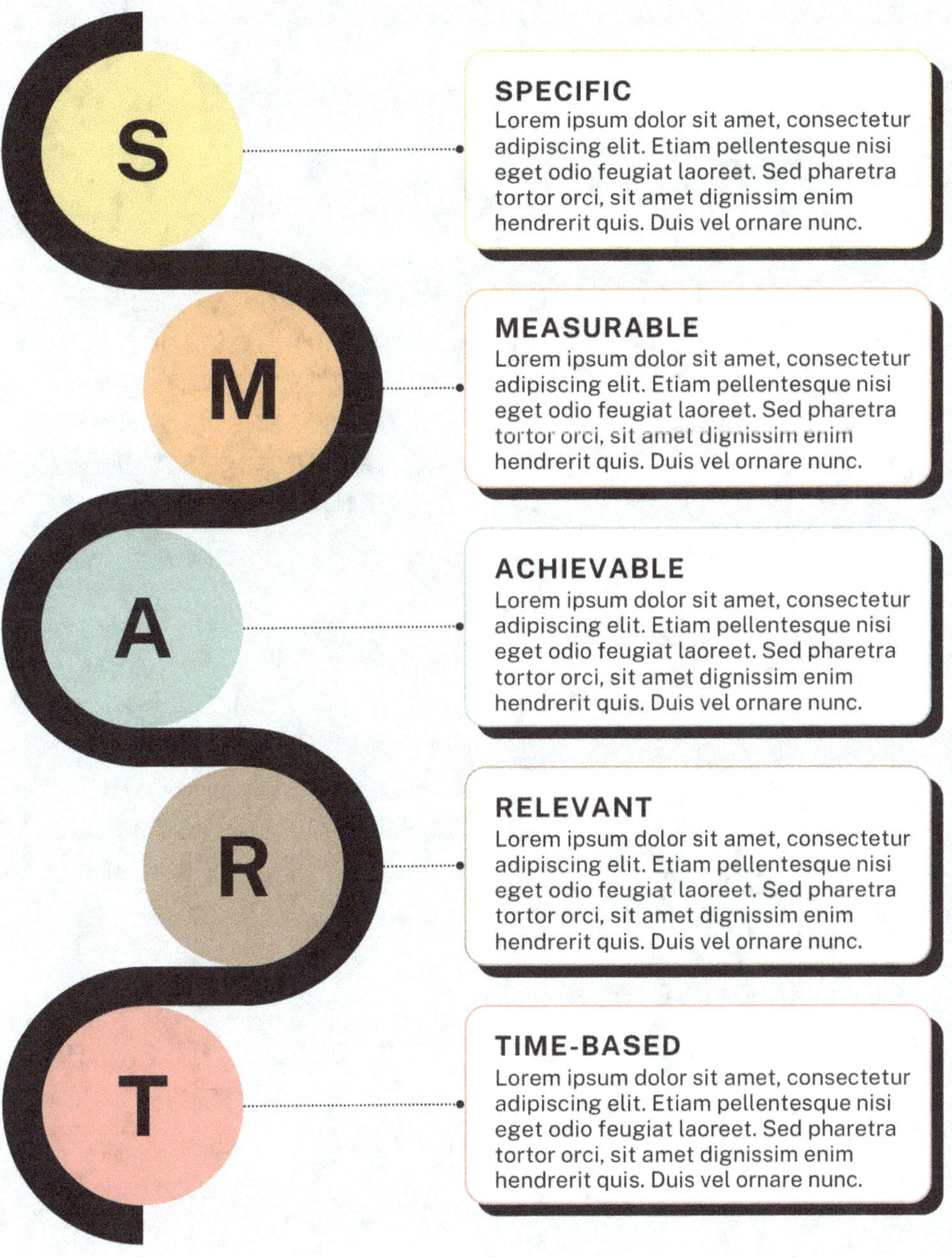

SMART

S

M

A

R

T

SPECIFIC
Lorem ipsum dolor sit amet, consectetur adipiscing elit. Etiam pellentesque nisi eget odio feugiat laoreet. Sed pharetra tortor orci, sit amet dignissim enim hendrerit quis. Duis vel ornare nunc.

MEASURABLE
Lorem ipsum dolor sit amet, consectetur adipiscing elit. Etiam pellentesque nisi eget odio feugiat laoreet. Sed pharetra tortor orci, sit amet dignissim enim hendrerit quis. Duis vel ornare nunc.

ACHIEVABLE
Lorem ipsum dolor sit amet, consectetur adipiscing elit. Etiam pellentesque nisi eget odio feugiat laoreet. Sed pharetra tortor orci, sit amet dignissim enim hendrerit quis. Duis vel ornare nunc.

RELEVANT
Lorem ipsum dolor sit amet, consectetur adipiscing elit. Etiam pellentesque nisi eget odio feugiat laoreet. Sed pharetra tortor orci, sit amet dignissim enim hendrerit quis. Duis vel ornare nunc.

TIME-BASED
Lorem ipsum dolor sit amet, consectetur adipiscing elit. Etiam pellentesque nisi eget odio feugiat laoreet. Sed pharetra tortor orci, sit amet dignissim enim hendrerit quis. Duis vel ornare nunc.

MENTAL <u>HEALTH</u>

TAKING CARE OF YOUR MENTAL HEALTH

PRACTICAL TIPS FOR EVERYDAY WELL-BEING

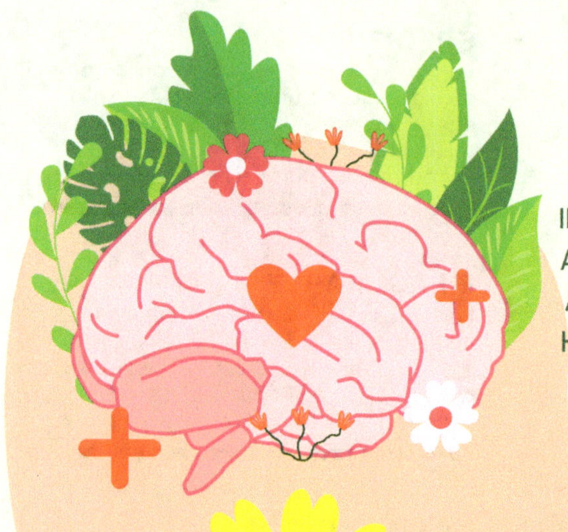

MENTAL HEALTH IS JUST AS IMPORTANT AS PHYSICAL HEALTH. IT AFFECTS HOW WE THINK, FEEL, AND ACT. TAKING CARE OF OUR MENTAL HEALTH IS ESSENTIAL FOR OVERALL WELL-BEING. HERE ARE SOME PRACTICAL TIPS TO HELP YOU MAINTAIN GOOD MENTAL HEALTH.

PRACTICE SELF-CARE. TAKE TIME TO DO THINGS THAT YOU ENJOY, SUCH AS READING A BOOK, TAKING A WALK, OR HAVING A RELAXING BATH. PRIORITIZING SELF-CARE CAN HELP REDUCE STRESS AND IMPROVE MOOD.

CONNECT WITH OTHERS. HAVING A SUPPORT SYSTEM IS CRUCIAL FOR GOOD MENTAL HEALTH. REACH OUT TO FRIENDS, FAMILY, OR A MENTAL HEALTH PROFESSIONAL IF YOU NEED TO TALK OR RECEIVE GUIDANCE.

Psychology center:
Discover the path to well-being

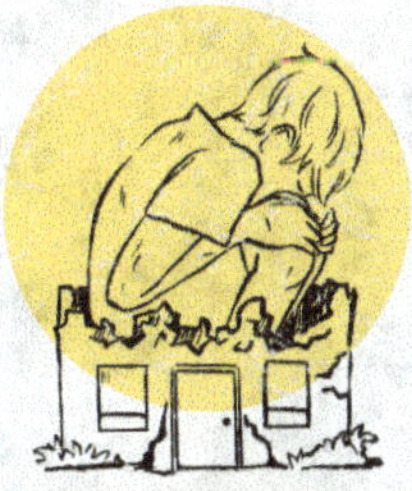

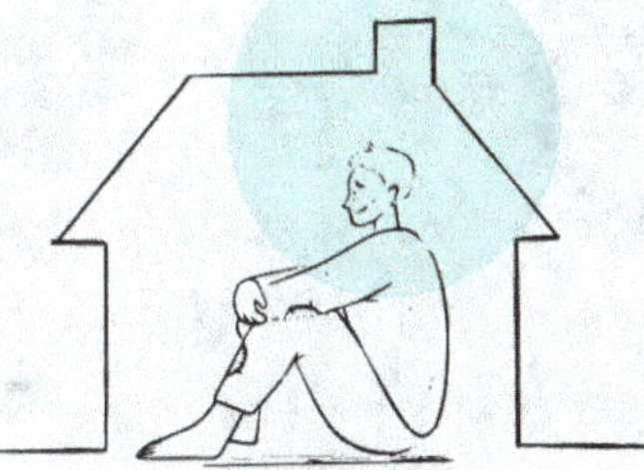

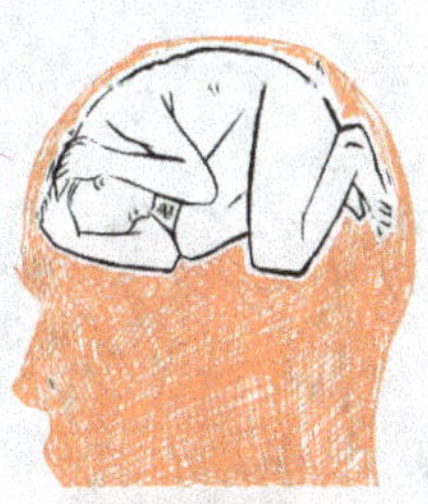

Individual therapy

Couples therapy

Well-being workshops

Lorem ipsum dolor sit amet, consectetur adipiscing elit, sed do eiusmod tempor incididunt ut labore et dolore magna aliqua. Ut enim ad minim veniam.

Lorem ipsum dolor sit amet, consectetur adipiscing elit, sed do eiusmod tempor incididunt ut labore et dolore magna aliqua. Ut enim ad minim veniam.

Lorem ipsum dolor sit amet, consectetur adipiscing elit, sed do eiusmod tempor incididunt ut labore et dolore magna aliqua. Ut enim ad minim veniam.

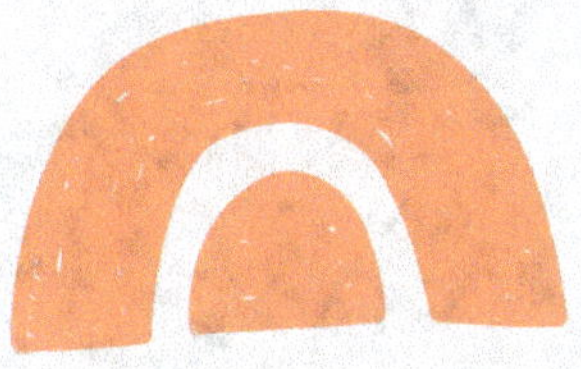

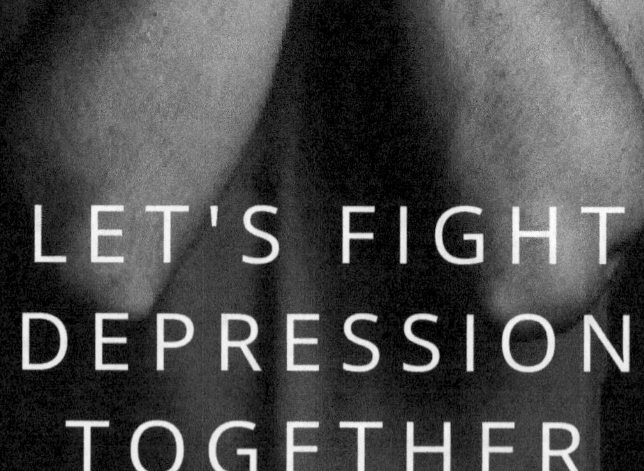
LET'S FIGHT
DEPRESSION
TOGETHER

"HEY LET'S TALK"

DON'T LET THEM SUFFER ALONE IN SILENCE.

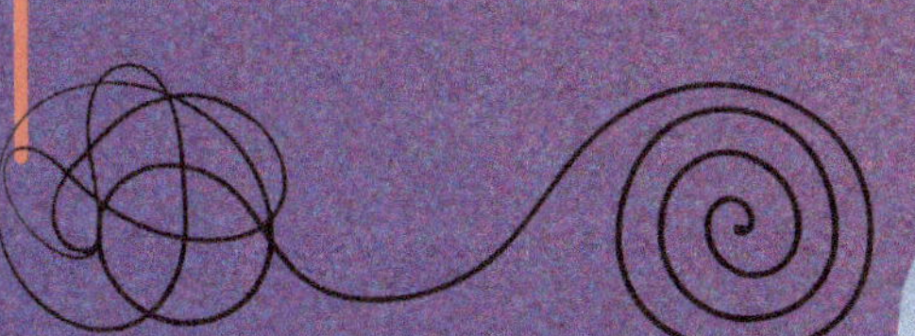

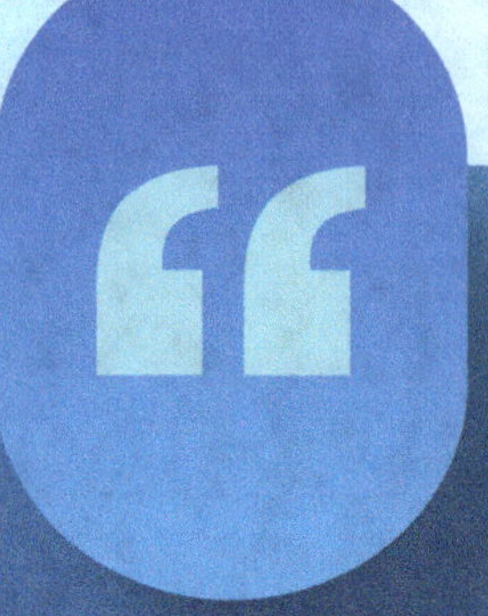

Do things at your **own** pace. Life is not a **race.**

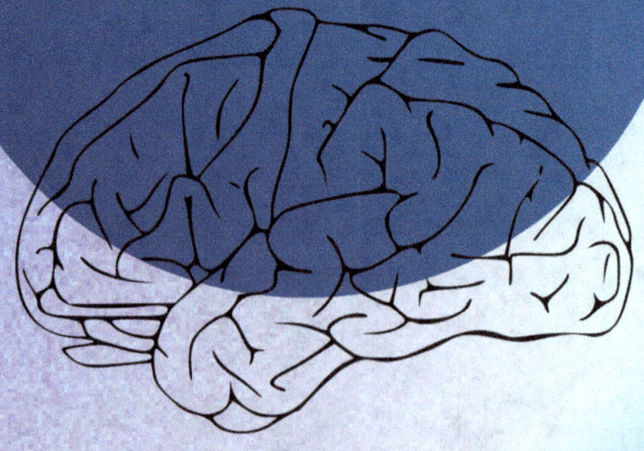

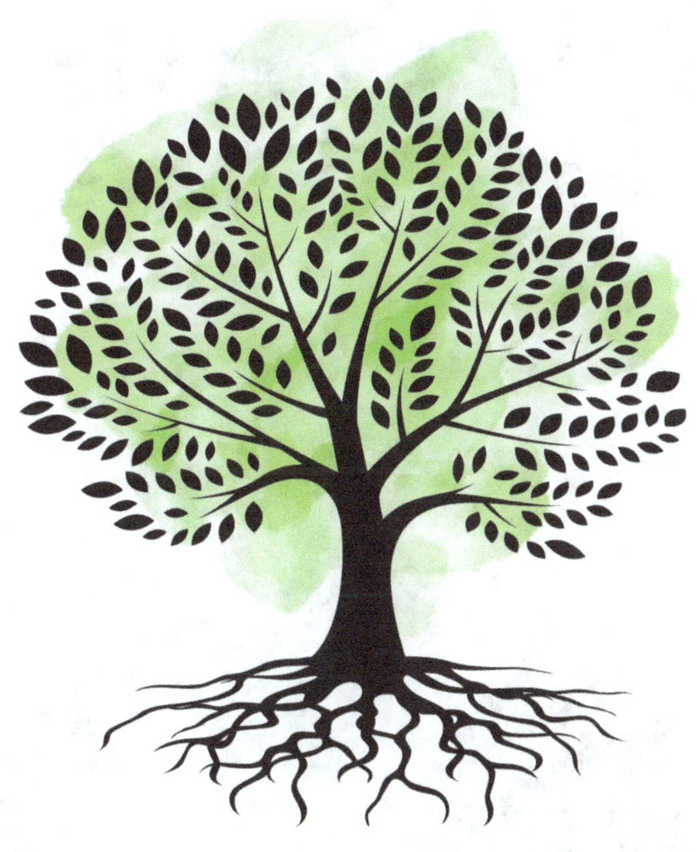

MINDFULNESS FOR MENTAL HEALTH

Cultivating awareness and inner peace

Mindfulness is the practice of being present and aware in the moment. It can help reduce stress and anxiety, improve mood, and promote overall well-being. Here are some tips to help you cultivate mindfulness.

Start with your breath. Take a few deep breaths and focus on the sensation of the air moving in and out of your body. This can help you become more grounded and present.

Practice mindful meditation. Set aside a few minutes each day to sit in quiet reflection. Focus on your breath, body sensations, or a mantra to help you stay present.

Engage your senses. Take a few moments to notice the sights, sounds, smells, and tastes around you. Engaging your senses can help bring you into the present moment.

Don't be afraid to ask for help

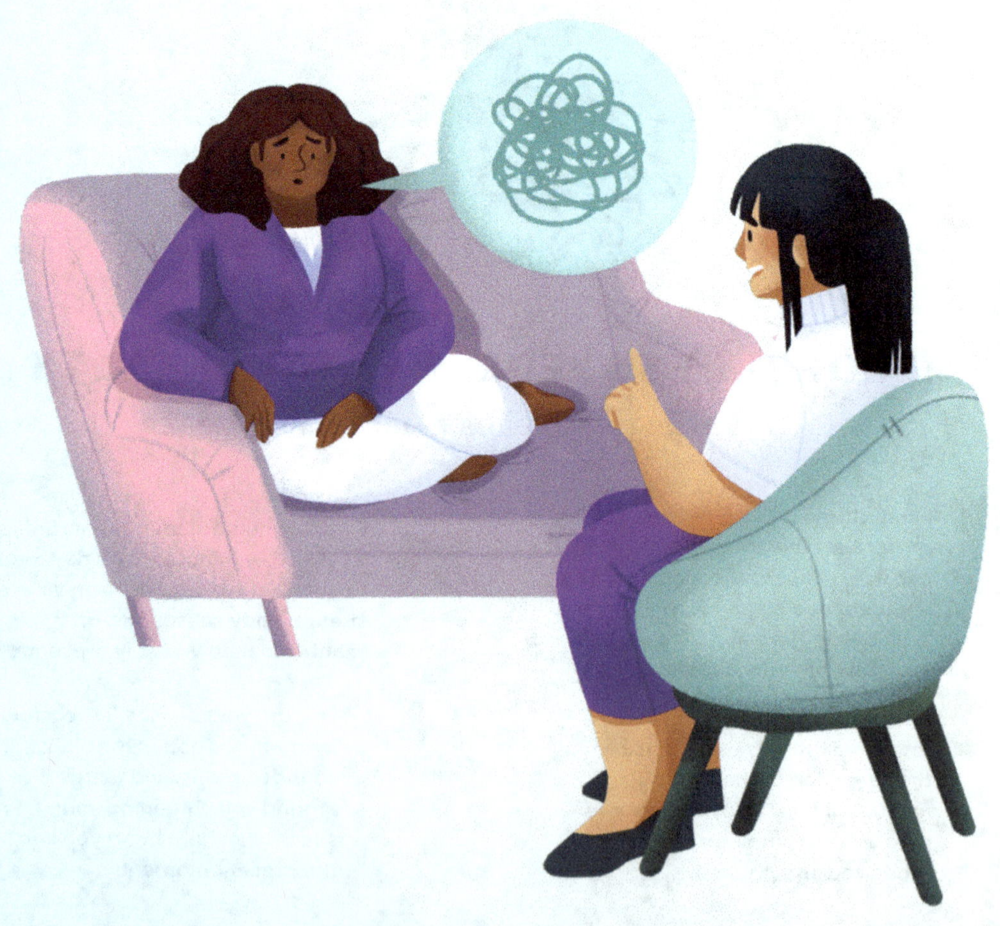

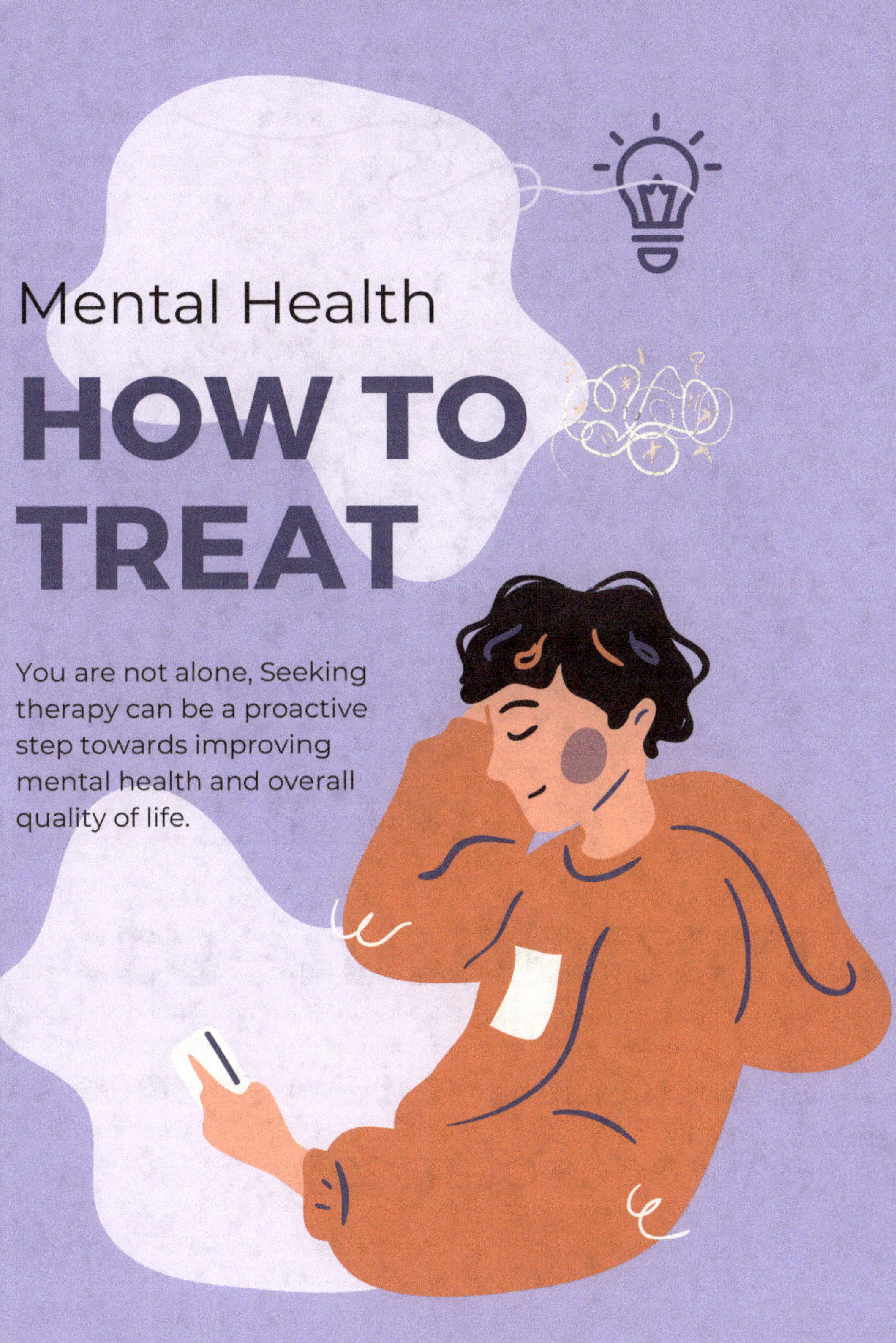

Mental Health
HOW TO TREAT
You are not alone, Seeking therapy can be a proactive step towards improving mental health and overall quality of life.

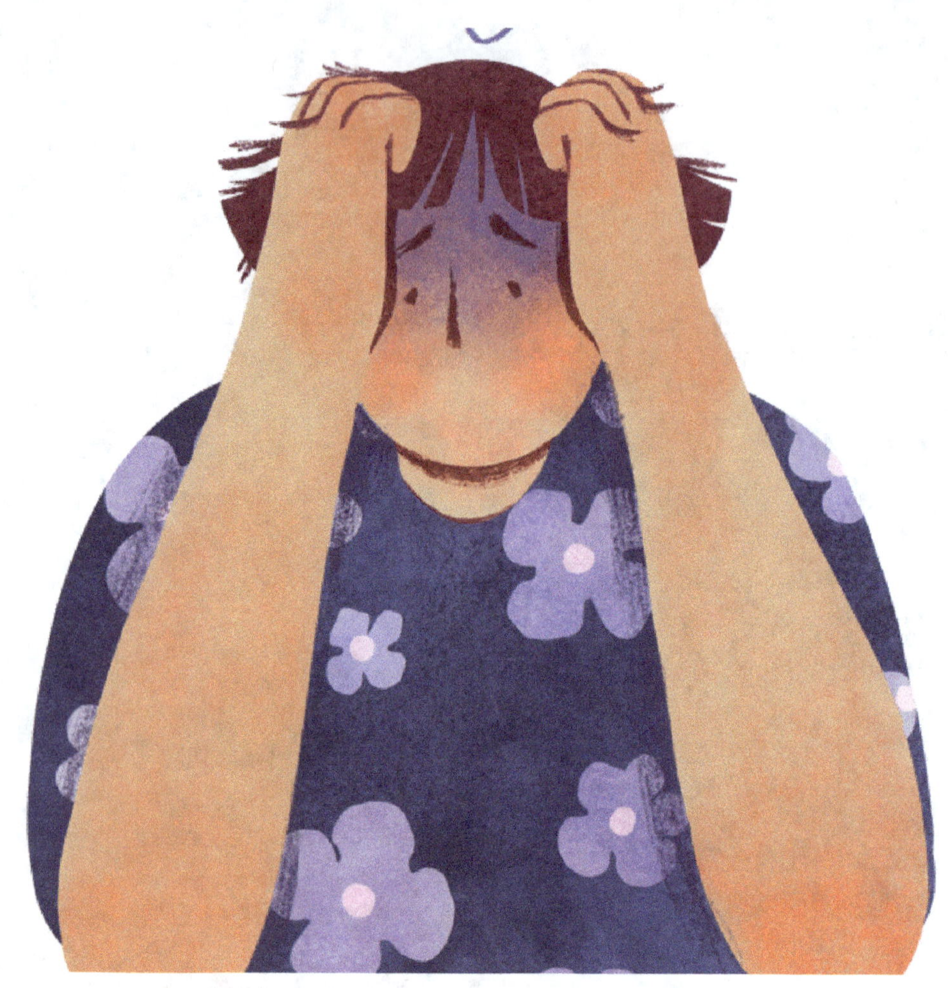

mindfulness:

the practice of awareness and acceptance

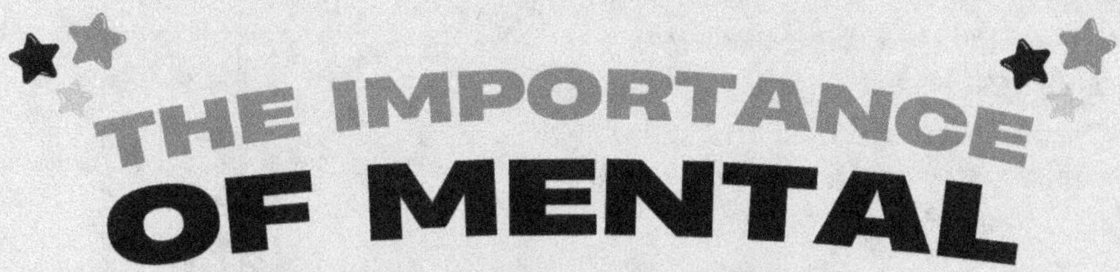

THE IMPORTANCE OF MENTAL

HEALTH AWARENESS

Mental health awareness helps reduce stigma, promotes empathy, and encourages open conversations about mental health concerns.

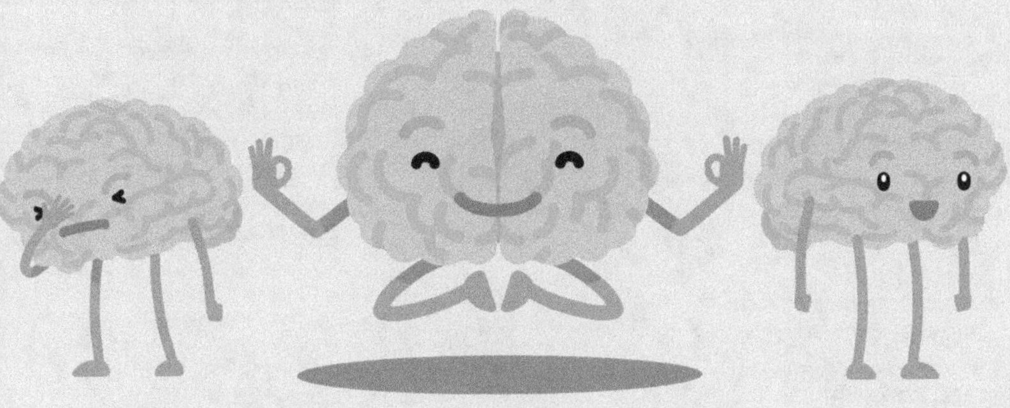

01

Increased mental health awareness leads to early recognition and intervention of mental health issues, improving outcomes and preventing further distress.

02

Mental health awareness helps reduce stigma, promotes empathy, and encourages open conversations about mental health concerns.

03

Mental health awareness involves understanding and recognizing the importance of mental well-being and the impact of mental health on overall quality of life.

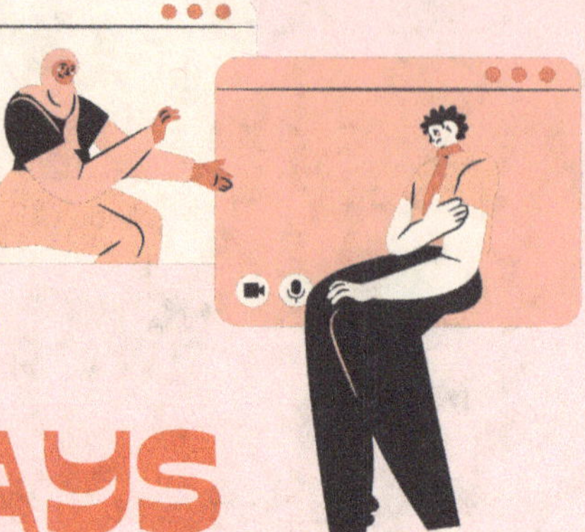

SIMPLE WAYS TO RELIEVE
Stress and Anxiety

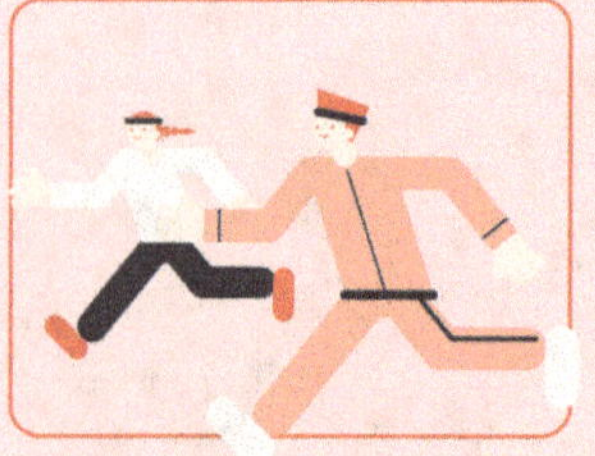

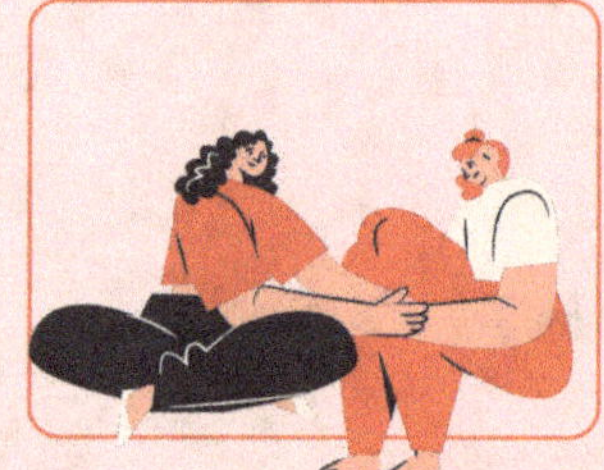

THE BENEFITS ARE STRONGEST WHEN YOU EXERCISE REGULARLY. PEOPLE WHO EXERCISE REGULARLY ARE LESS LIKELY TO EXPERIENCE ANXIETY THAN THOSE WHO DON'T EXERCISE.

02

USING ESSENTIAL OILS OR BURNING A SCENTED CANDLE MAY HELP REDUCE YOUR FEELINGS OF STRESS AND ANXIETY.

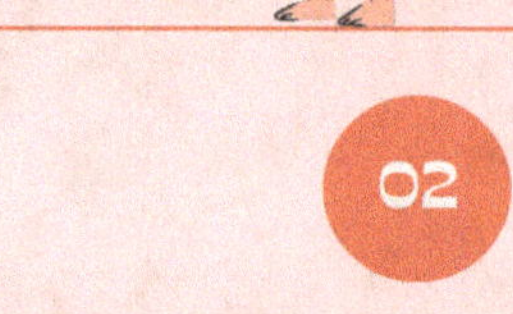

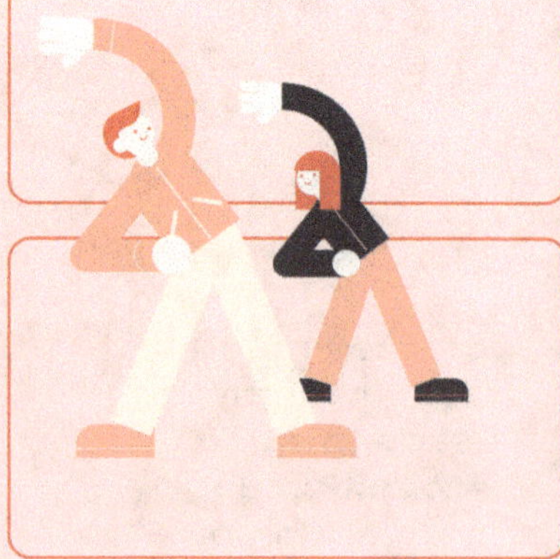

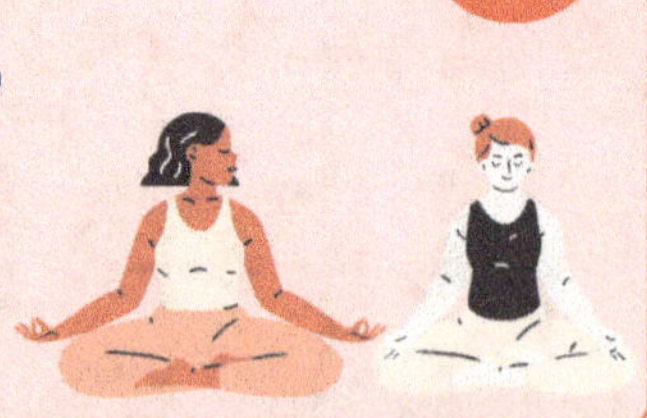

03

REACH OUT TO TRUSTED FRIENDS, FAMILY MEMBERS, OR SUPPORT GROUPS. SHARING YOUR FEELINGS AND CONCERNS WITH OTHERS CAN PROVIDE COMFORT AND PERSPECTIVE.

04

ENGAGE IN ACTIVITIES YOU ENJOY, SUCH AS READING, LISTENING TO MUSIC, PAINTING, OR PRACTICING A HOBBY. TAKING TIME FOR YOURSELF AND DOING THINGS YOU LOVE CAN HELP REDUCE STRESS.

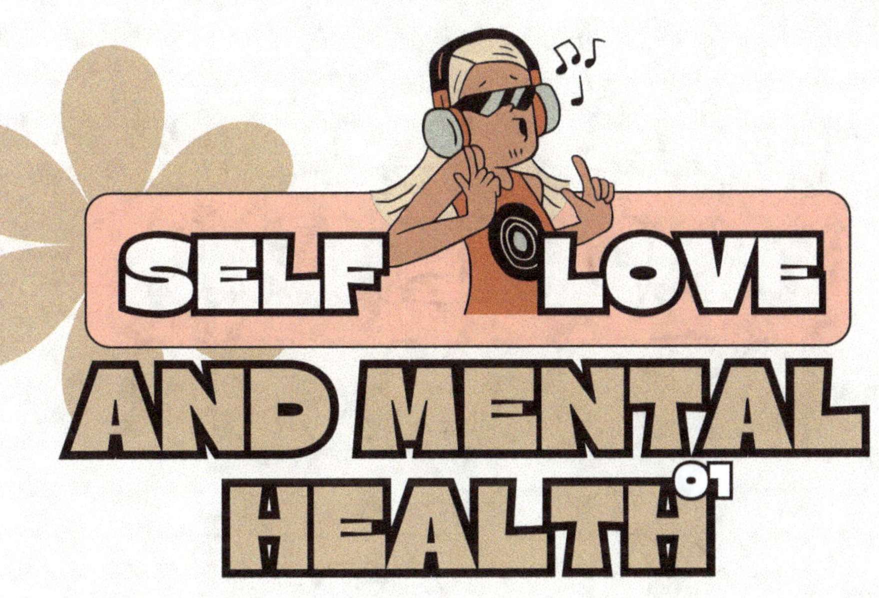

SELF LOVE AND MENTAL HEALTH [01]

01

Self-love is a practice of nurturing and valuing oneself. It includes accepting both strengths and weaknesses and prioritizing self-care.

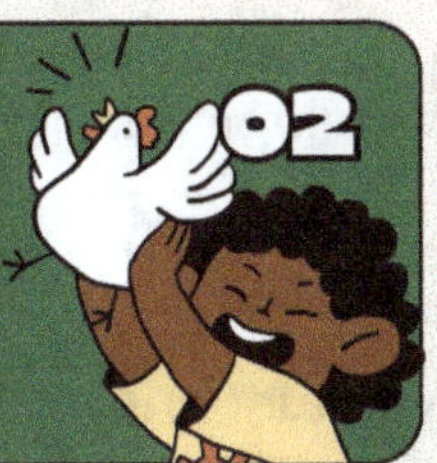

02

Practicing self-love can improve mental health by boosting self-esteem, self-confidence, and resilience in the face of challenges.

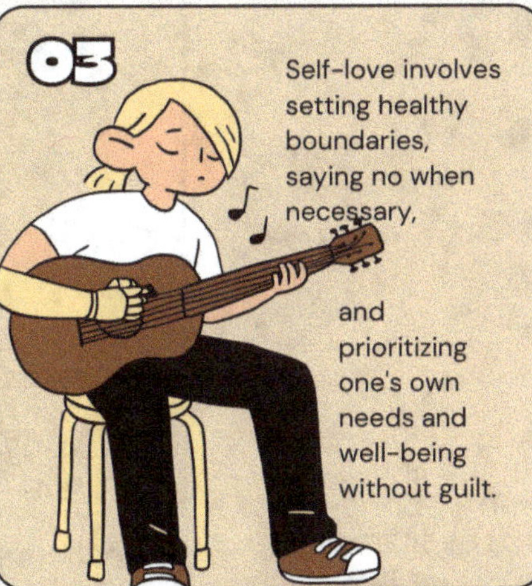

03

Self-love involves setting healthy boundaries, saying no when necessary,

and prioritizing one's own needs and well-being without guilt.

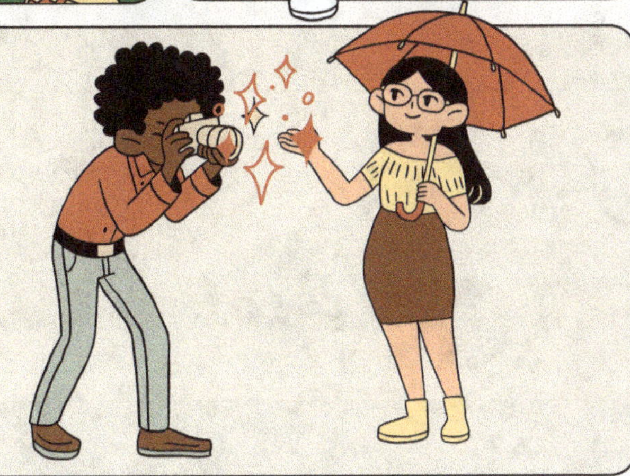

Self-love includes practicing self-compassion and treating oneself with kindness and understanding during difficult times or when facing setbacks.

04

BUILDING RESILIENCE AND MENTAL STRENGTH

01

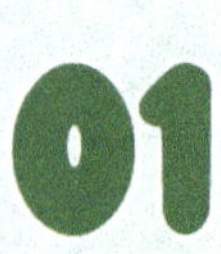

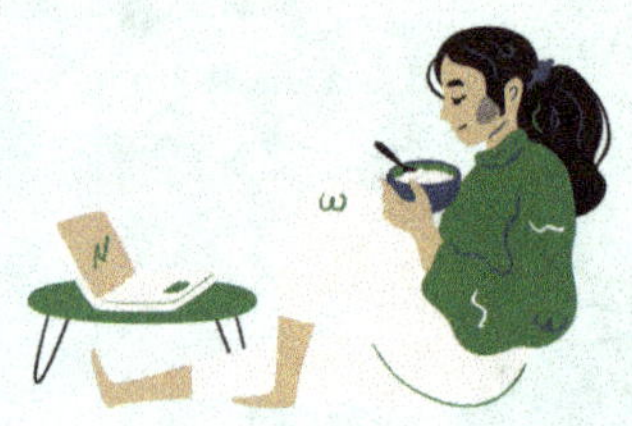

Resilience is the ability to adapt, bounce back, and recover from adversity, trauma, or significant life challenges

02

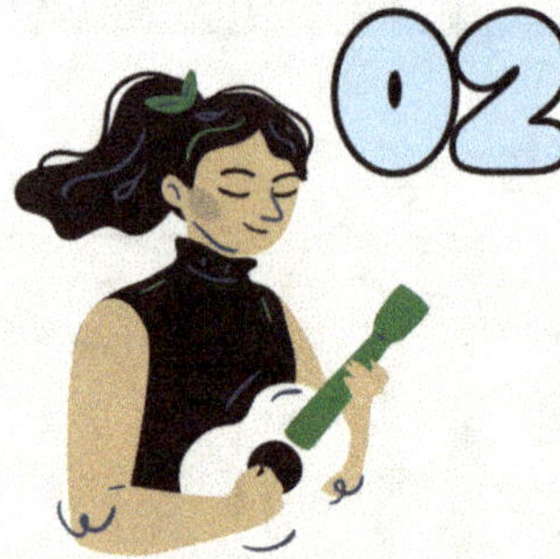

Building resilience involves developing a positive mindset, focusing on strengths, and cultivating optimism even in challenging situations.

Resilience can be nurtured through self-care practices. You can exercise, get enough sleep, healthy eating, and engage in activities that bring joy and relaxation.

03

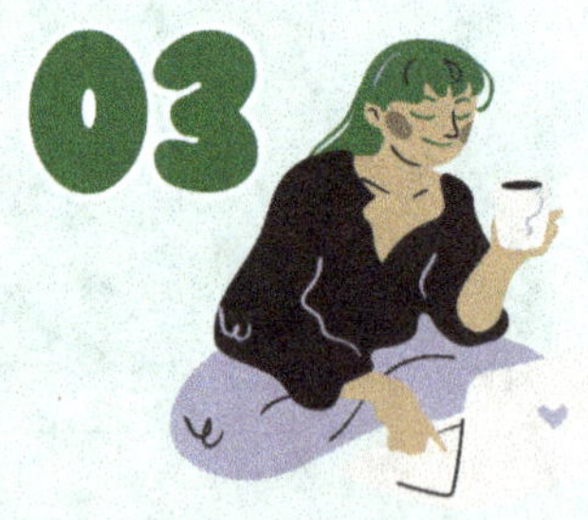

04

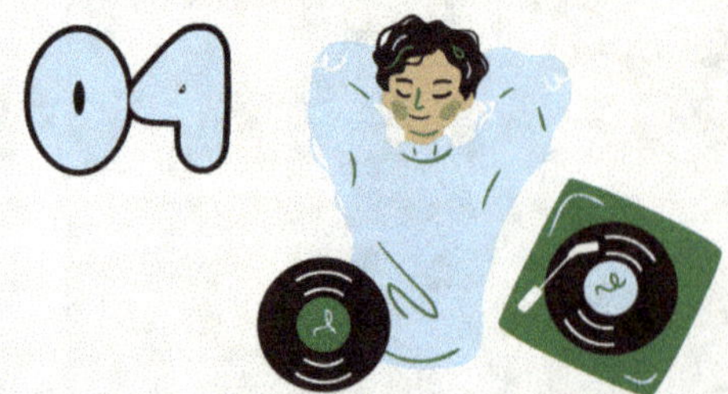

Building a strong support system with friends, family, or support groups can enhance resilience by providing emotional support, understanding, and encouragement.

STRESS MANAGEMENT

ON THE PATH TO INNER PEACE

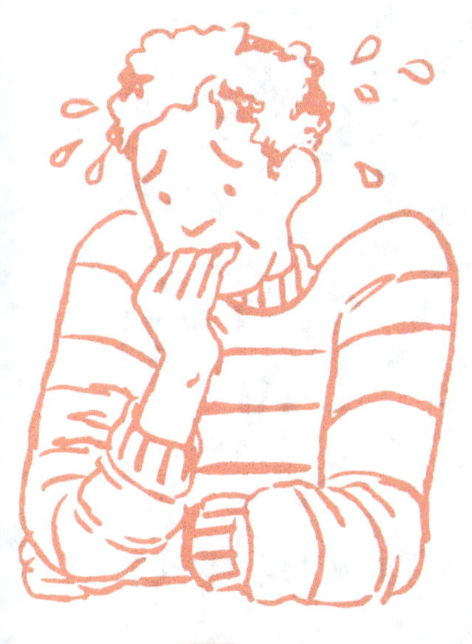

Explore new stress coping techniques to find inner serenity

Understand how stress impacts psychology and physiology, and discover healthy ways to cope with it

Learn relaxation and meditation methods to reduce tension and anxiety

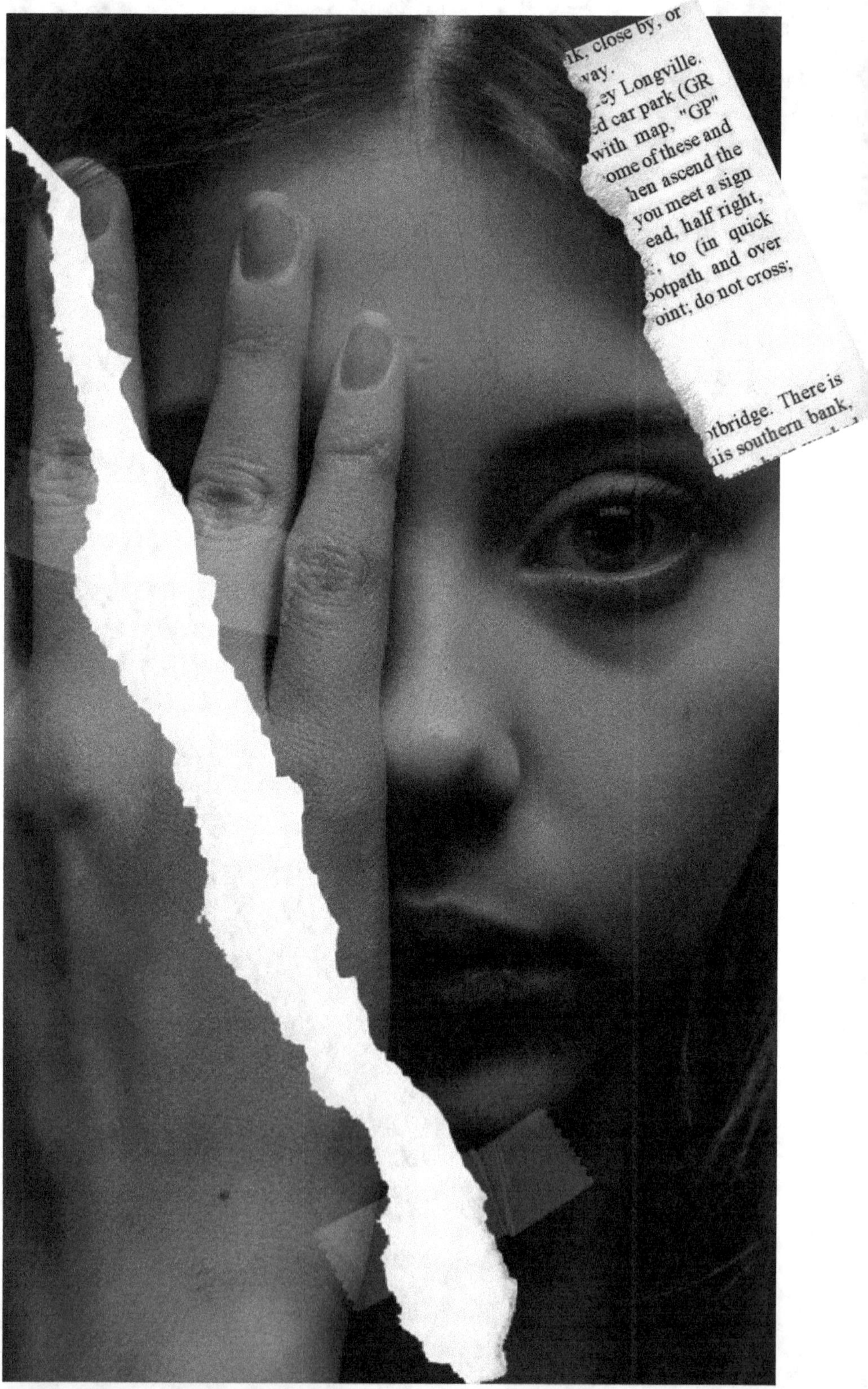

nk, close by, or
vay.
ey Longville.
d car park (GR
with map, "GP"
ome of these and
hen ascend the
you meet a sign
ead, half right,
to (in quick
otpath and over
oint; do not cross;

otbridge. There is
is southern bank,

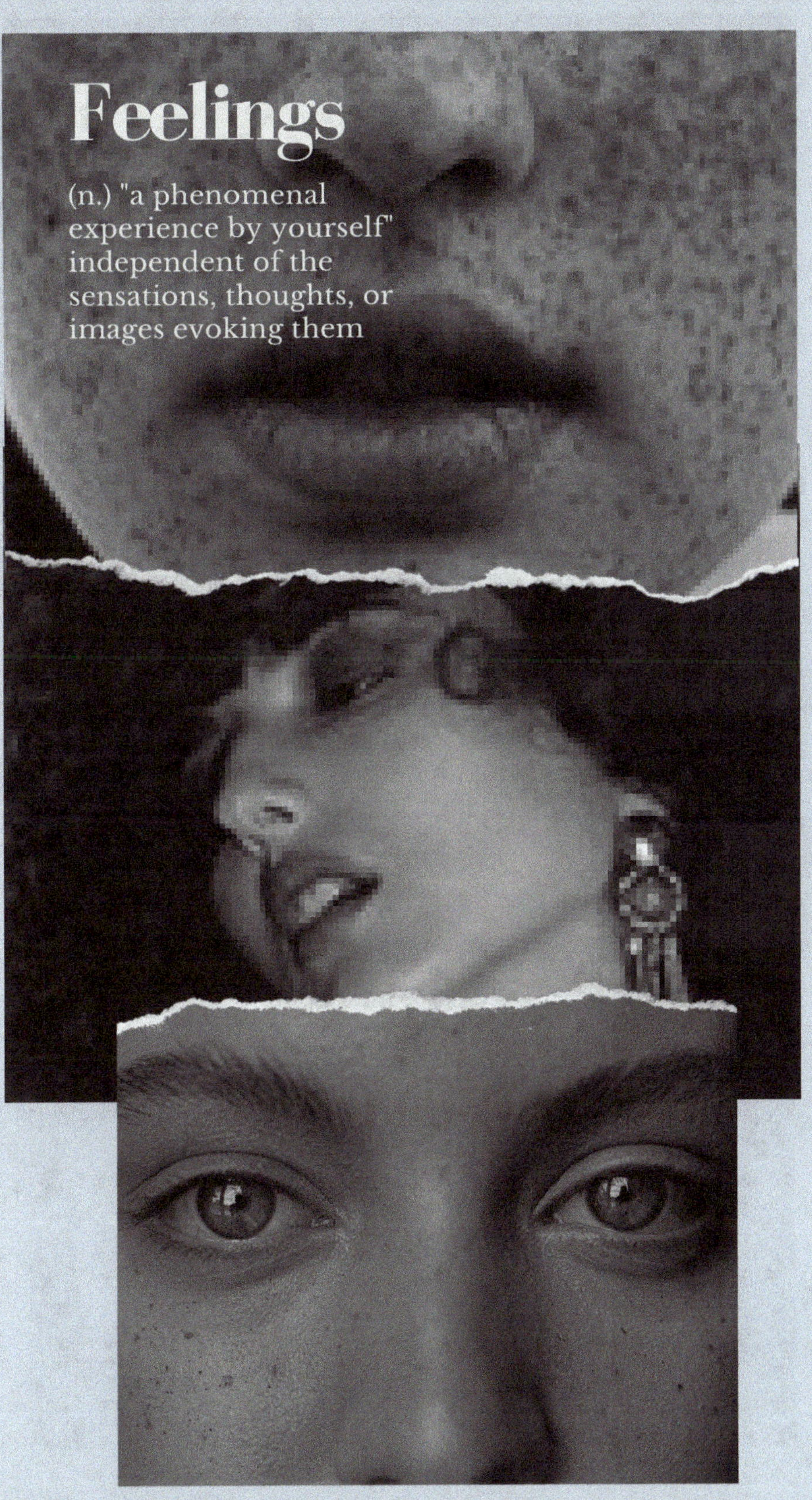

Feelings
(n.) "a phenomenal experience by yourself" independent of the sensations, thoughts, or images evoking them

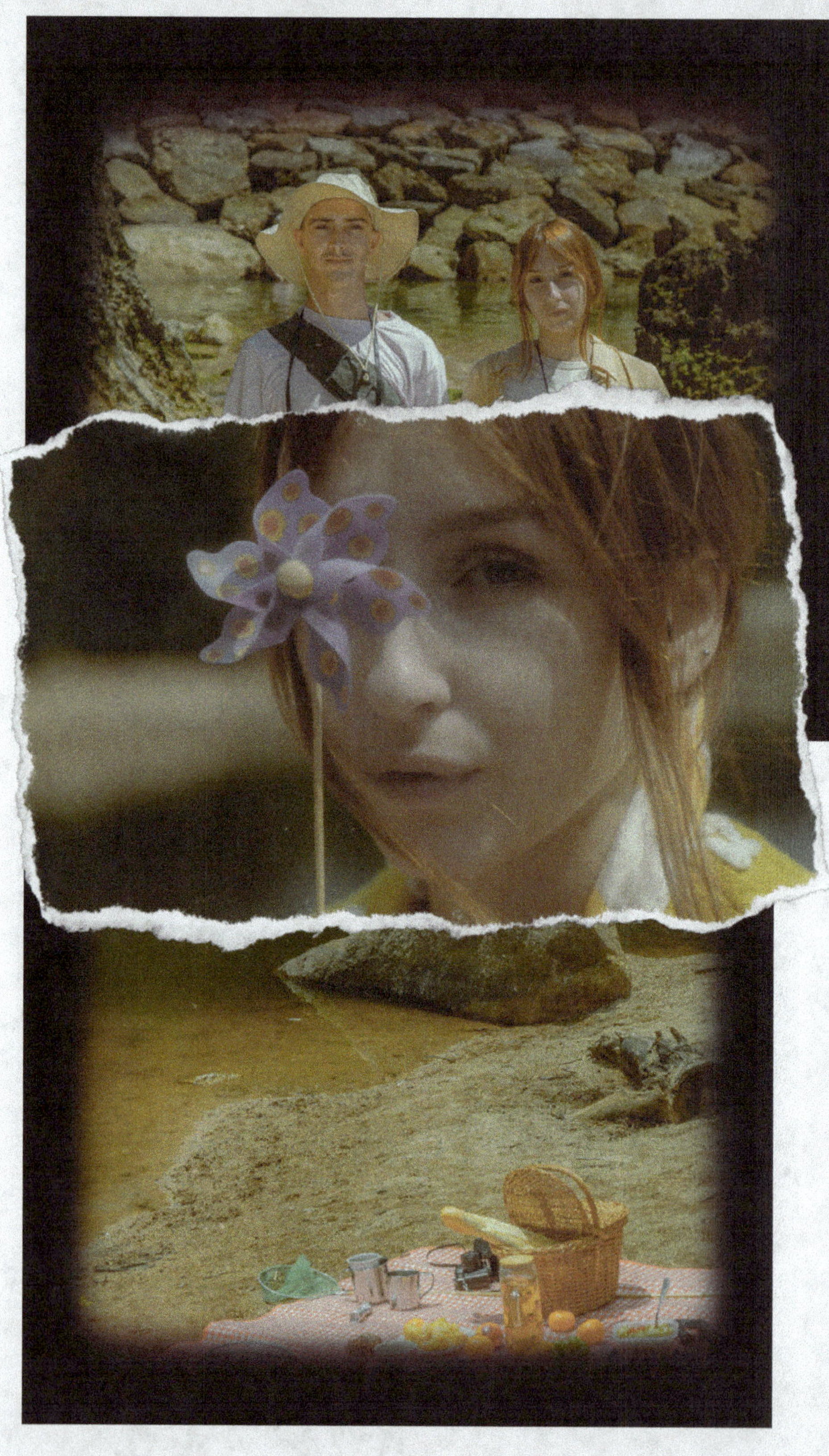

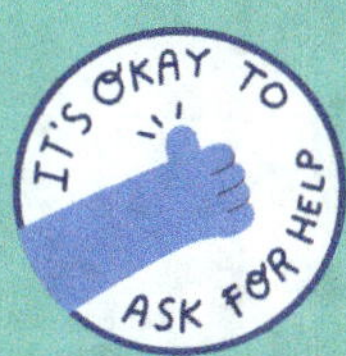

PRIORITIZING
MENTAL HEALTH

01

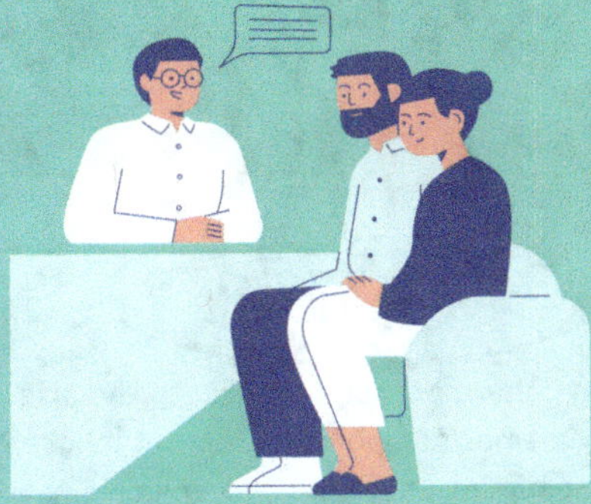

Seek support from trusted individuals or professionals

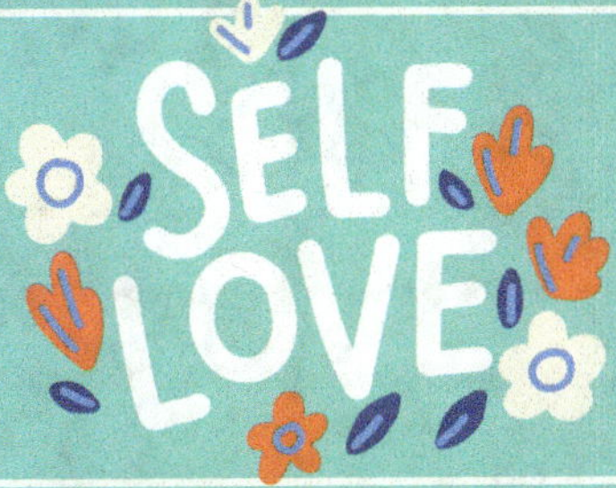

02

Engage in activities that promote relaxation and self-care.

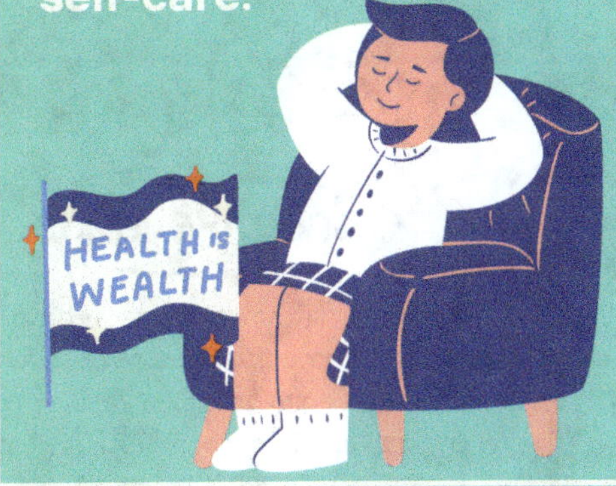

03

Practice stress reduction techniques, such as journaling or talking openly about emotions.

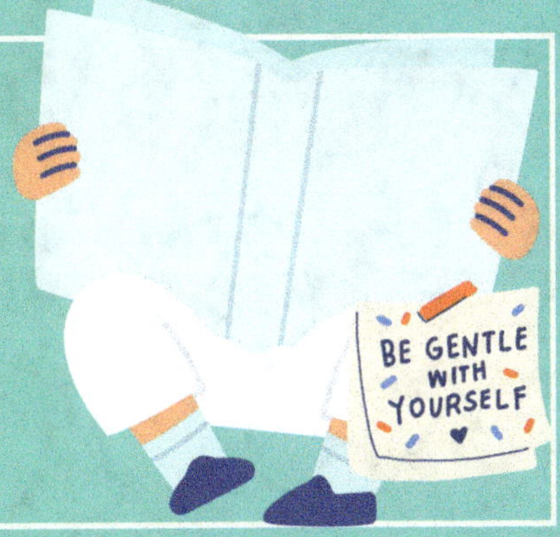

The artistic
PROCESS

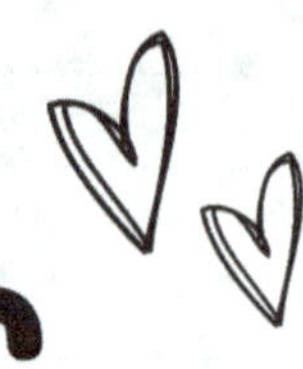

01

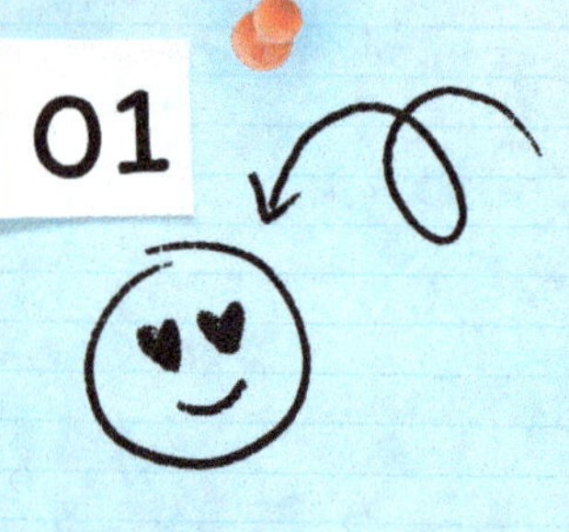

The artist

Lorem ipsum dolor sit amet, consectetur adipiscing elit, sed do eiusmod tempor incididunt ut labore et dolore magna aliqua. Ut enim ad minim veniam, quis nostrud exercitation ullamco laboris nisi ut aliquip ex ea commodo consequat.

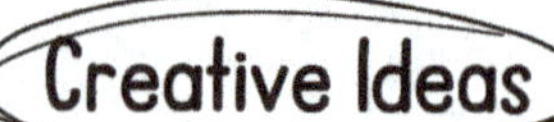

Creative Ideas

Lorem ipsum dolor sit amet, consectetur adipiscing elit, sed do eiusmod tempor incididunt ut labore et dolore magna aliqua. Ut enim ad minim veniam, quis nostrud exercitation ullamco laboris nisi ut aliquip ex ea commodo consequat.

02

03

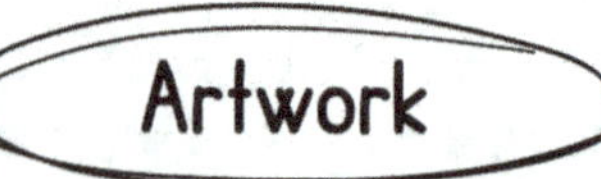

Artwork

Lorem ipsum dolor sit amet, consectetur adipiscing elit, sed do eiusmod tempor incididunt ut labore et dolore magna aliqua. Ut enim ad minim veniam, quis nostrud exercitation ullamco laboris nisi ut aliquip ex ea commodo consequat.

Learn to manage emotions

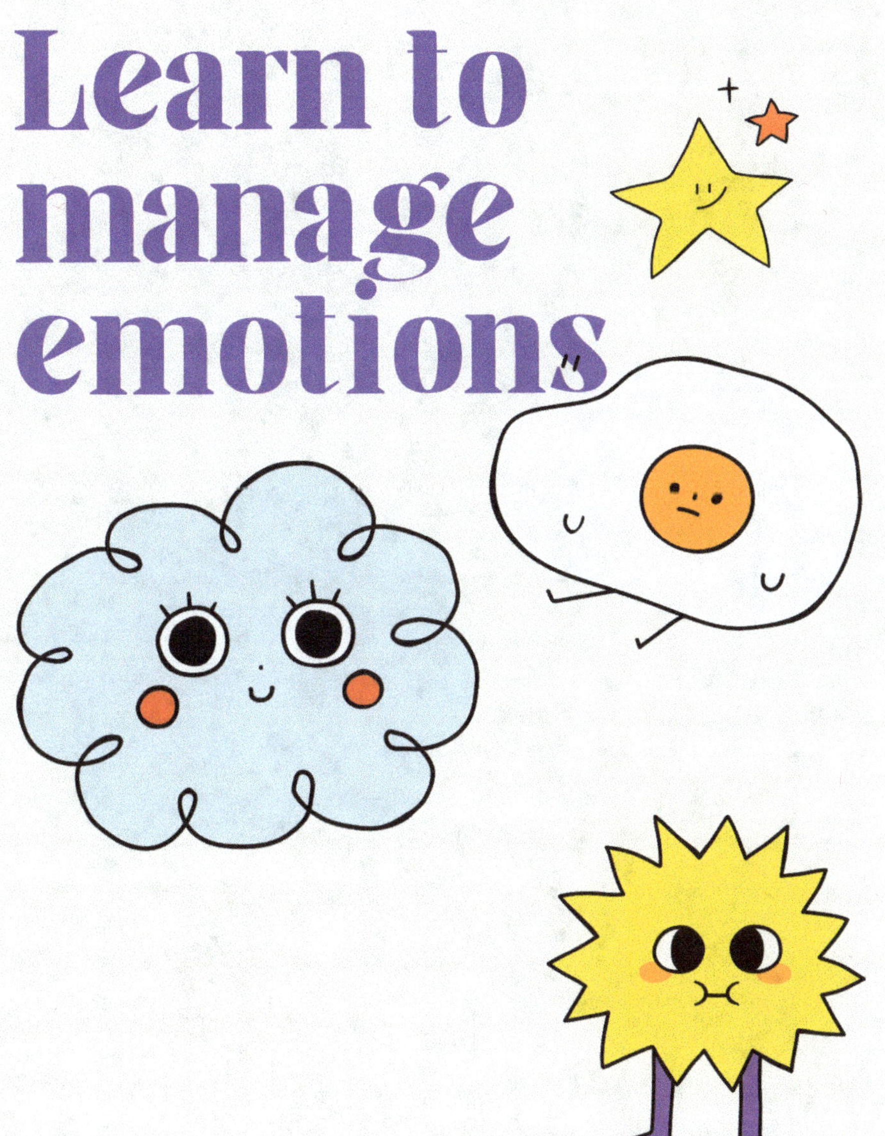

Self Care

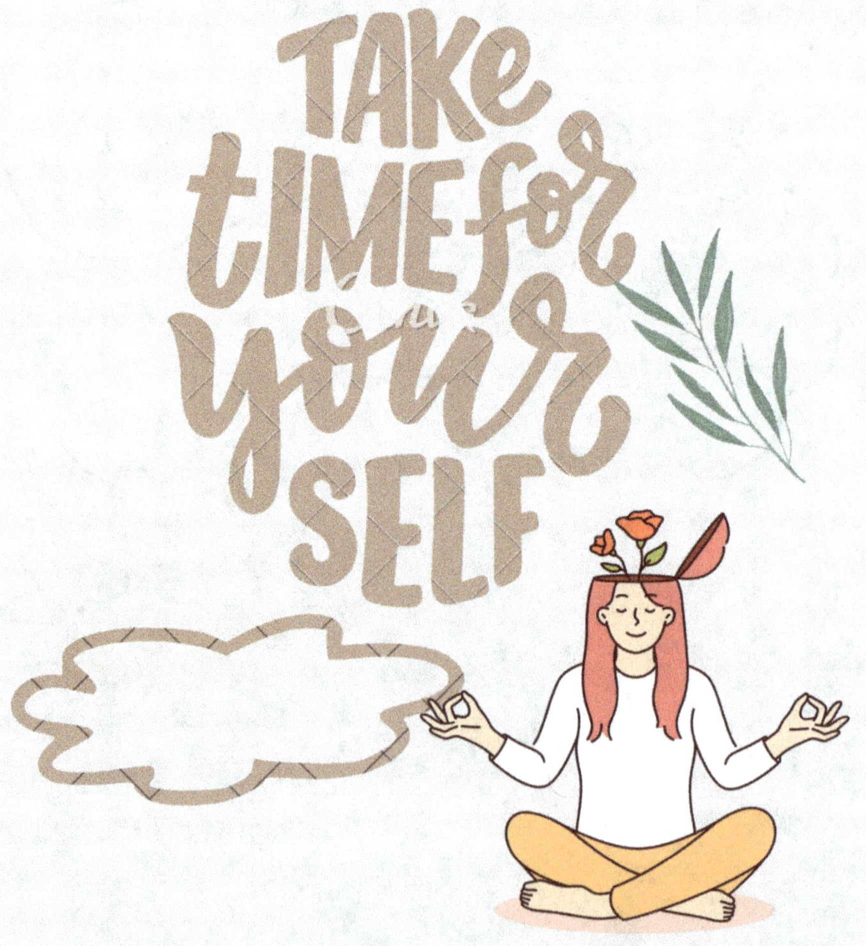

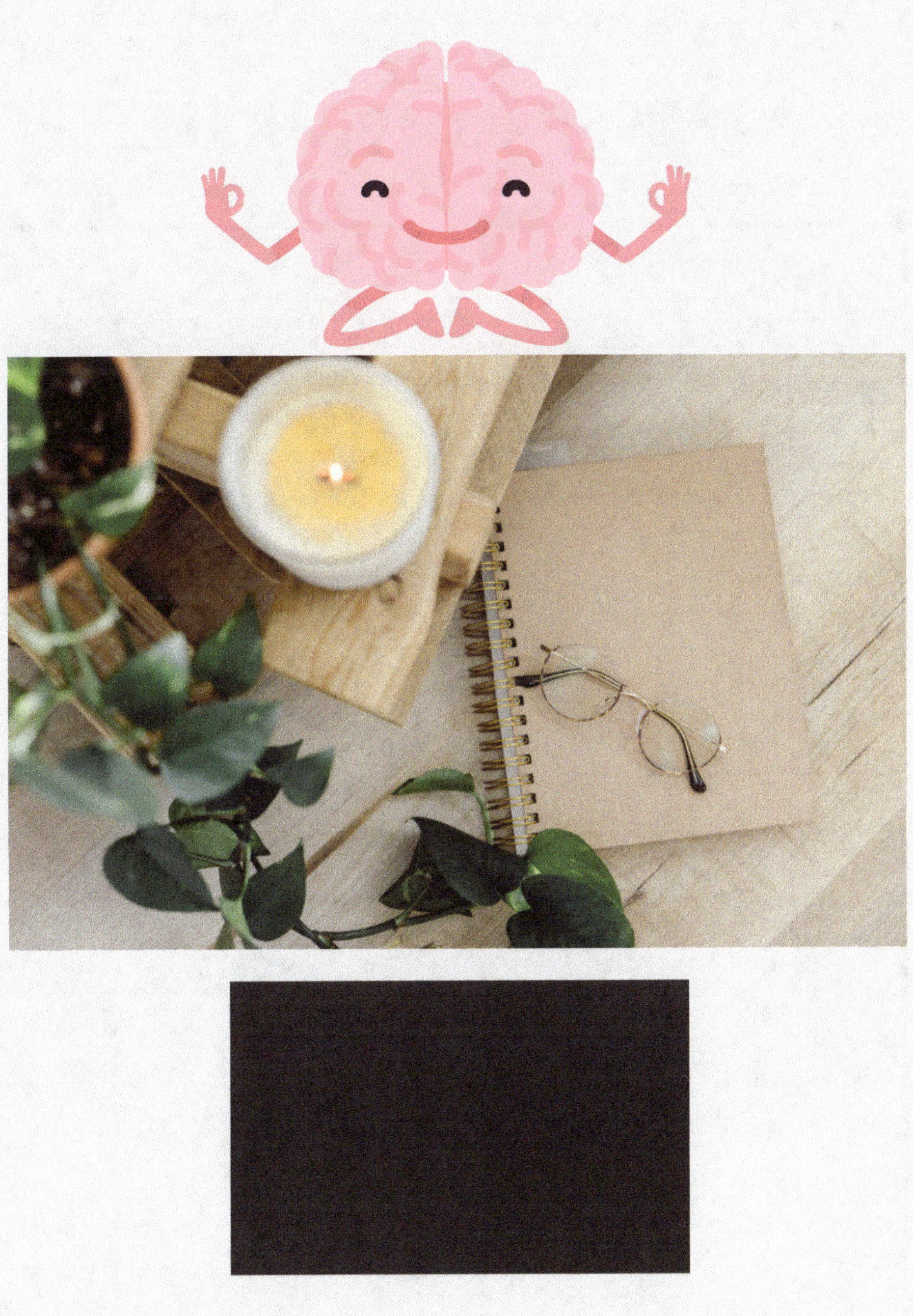

ASSESSING YOURSELF

Physical Self Care

	Y	N
Got Enough Sleep	○	○
Eat healthy	○	○
Balanced Diet	○	○
Get Regular Exercise	○	○
See a Healthcare Provider when needed	○	○

NOTE:

Mental Self Care

	Y	N
Take time to relax	○	○
Joy and Fulfillment in activities	○	○
Support System	○	○
Practice Mindfullness	○	○
Stay present in the moment	○	○

NOTE:

Social Self Care

	Y	N
Strong and Supportive Relationship with friends and family	○	○
Make time for social activity	○	○
Set Boundaries	○	○
Say no when necessary	○	○

NOTE:

Spiritual Self Care

	Y	N
Have a sense of purpose and meaning in your life	○	○
Practice self-reflection and mindfulness	○	○
Have a sense of connection to something larger than yourself	○	○

NOTE:

SELF-CARE IN PRACTICE

Effective stress management can be incorporated into your daily and weekly routines. Research has shown that the following can affect your health and well-being: Relaxation Skills, Food Choices, Physical Activity, and Spirituality/Connection. Write down options that seem right for you, your values, priorities, resources, and lifestyle.

RELAXATION PRACTICE	DIFFICULT FOR ME

FOOD CHOICES	DIFFICULT FOR ME

PHYSICAL ACTIVITY	DIFFICULT FOR ME

CONNECTION/SPIRITUALITY	DIFFICULT FOR ME

SEEKING SUPPORT

Seeking support when you're feeling overwhelmed or struggling with your mental or emotional well-being is essential. There are many different ways to find help, including:

1. Talk to a loved one: Sharing your feelings with a trusted friend or family can be a great way to find support. They can listen, offer advice, and be there for you when you need someone to talk to.
2. See a therapist: A therapist can help you work through your emotions and challenges in a safe and supportive environment. You can find therapists in your area by searching online directories or through your insurance provider.
3. Join a support group: Support groups are a great way to connect with others who are going through similar experiences. You can find support groups in your area by searching online or through local organizations.
4. Reach out to a helpline: Many helplines available can provide support and resources if you're feeling overwhelmed or struggling with your mental health.

Remember, it's okay to ask for help when you need it. Seeking support is a sign of strength and can be essential in taking care of yourself.

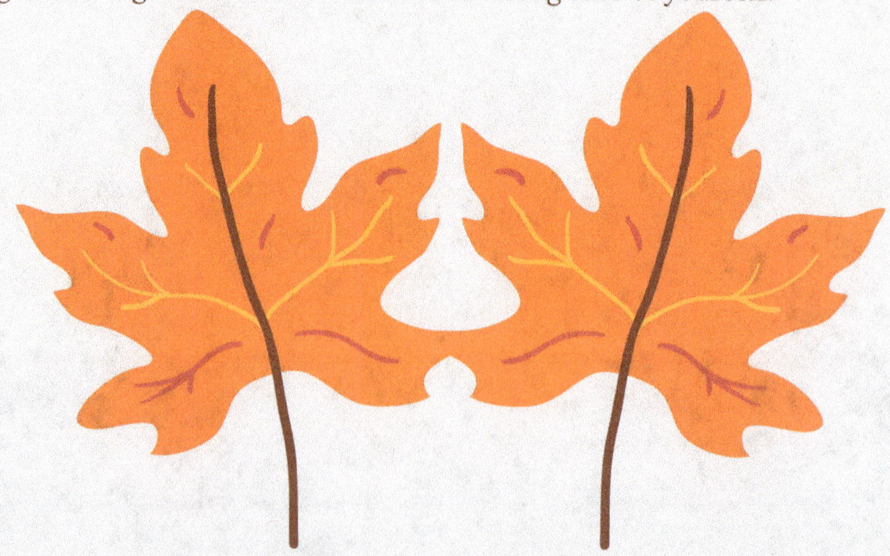

SELF-CARE CHECKLIST

Self-care isn't an act but a loving commitment to oneself.
How did you cherish yourself this week?

- ☐ Take a long bath
- ☐ Read for pleasure
- ☐ Go for a long walk
- ☐ Practice mindful meditation
- ☐ Journal your thoughts
- ☐ Try gentle yoga
- ☐ Cook a nourishing meal
- ☐ Visit a museum or gallery
- ☐ Gardening
- ☐ Paint or draw

- ☐ Engage in a hobby
- ☐ Listen to your favorite music
- ☐ Spend time with a loved one
- ☐ Watch a light-hearted movie
- ☐ Pamper yourself
- ☐ Take a short nap
- ☐ Go for a swim
- ☐ Practice gratitude
- ☐ Attend a workshop or class
- ☐ Explore a new place

WEEKLY
Cleaning Checklist

Everyday

- ○ wash dishes
- ○ make bed
- ○ take out trash
- ○ wipe down kitchen counters
- ○ vacuum
- ○ laundry

Monday (kitchen + dining room)

- ○ wipe down outside of fridge
- ○ wipe down sink, counters, table
- ○ spot clean cabinets
- ○ clean microwave
- ○ wipe down appliances and stove
- ○ clean windows
- ○ wipe down highchair
- ○ sweep and mop

Tuesday (living + playroom)

- ○ wipe down all counters
- ○ remove the dust
- ○ restock diaper
- ○ clean windows
- ○ organize kids toys
- ○ disinfect toys
- ○ tidy up the books

Wednesday (bathroom)

- ○ wipe down mirrors
- ○ clean toilets
- ○ clean showers and bathtubs
- ○ straighten inside of cabinets
- ○ empty trash
- ○ wash towels
- ○ shake out bath mats
- ○ sweep and mop

Thursday (bedroom)

- ○ wipe down night stands
- ○ remove the dust
- ○ straighten closet and dresser
- ○ wipe down window
- ○ wash bed linens
- ○ organize skincare products

Friday (random)

- ○ straighten laundry room
- ○ iron clothing
- ○ fold and put away laundry
- ○ disinfect shower curtains
- ○ wipe down washer and dryer
- ○ straighten craft area
- ○ organize the shoe closet

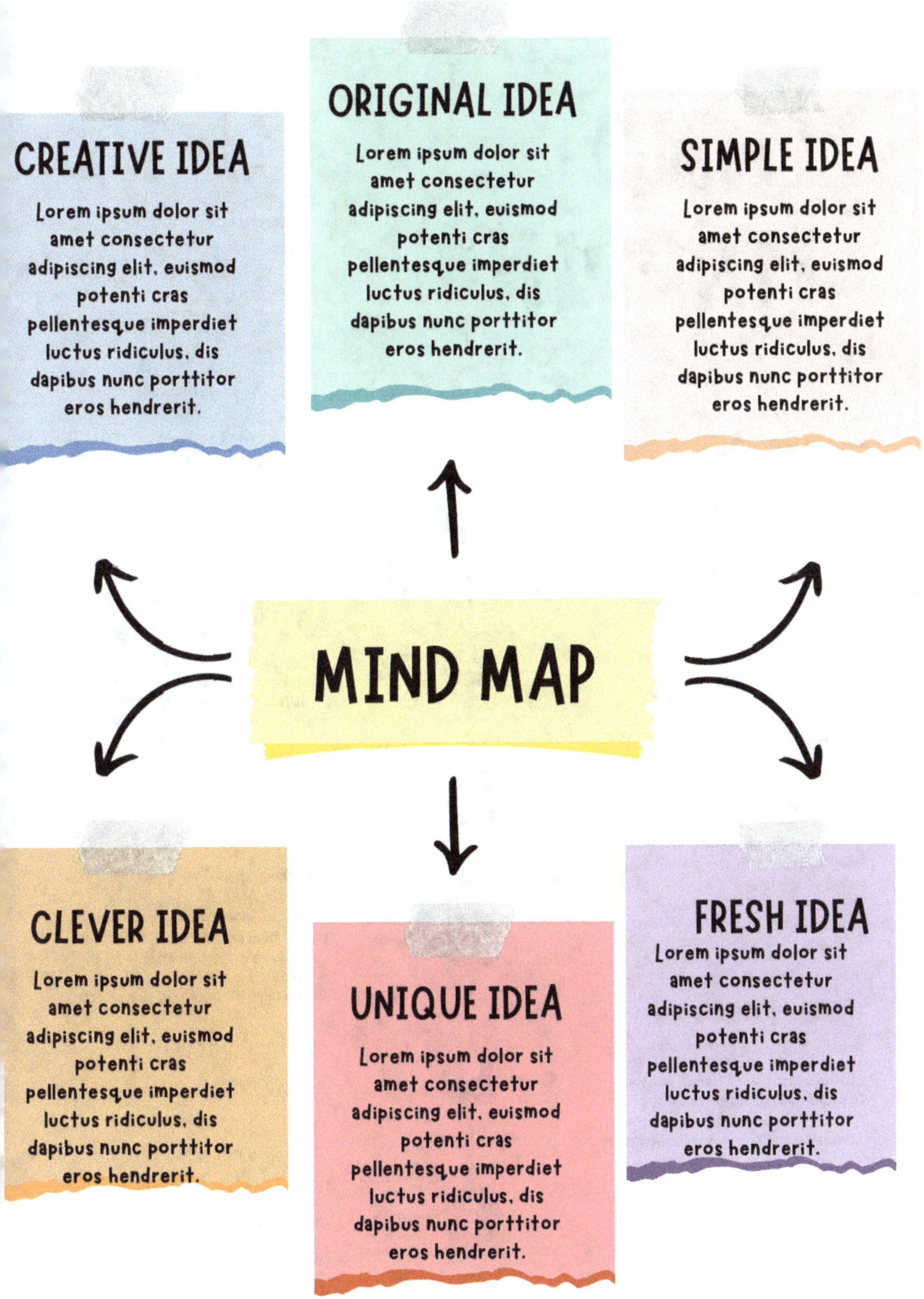

CREATIVE IDEA

Lorem ipsum dolor sit amet consectetur adipiscing elit, euismod potenti cras pellentesque imperdiet luctus ridiculus, dis dapibus nunc porttitor eros hendrerit.

ORIGINAL IDEA

Lorem ipsum dolor sit amet consectetur adipiscing elit, euismod potenti cras pellentesque imperdiet luctus ridiculus, dis dapibus nunc porttitor eros hendrerit.

SIMPLE IDEA

Lorem ipsum dolor sit amet consectetur adipiscing elit, euismod potenti cras pellentesque imperdiet luctus ridiculus, dis dapibus nunc porttitor eros hendrerit.

MIND MAP

CLEVER IDEA

Lorem ipsum dolor sit amet consectetur adipiscing elit, euismod potenti cras pellentesque imperdiet luctus ridiculus, dis dapibus nunc porttitor eros hendrerit.

UNIQUE IDEA

Lorem ipsum dolor sit amet consectetur adipiscing elit, euismod potenti cras pellentesque imperdiet luctus ridiculus, dis dapibus nunc porttitor eros hendrerit.

FRESH IDEA

Lorem ipsum dolor sit amet consectetur adipiscing elit, euismod potenti cras pellentesque imperdiet luctus ridiculus, dis dapibus nunc porttitor eros hendrerit.

MIND MAPPING

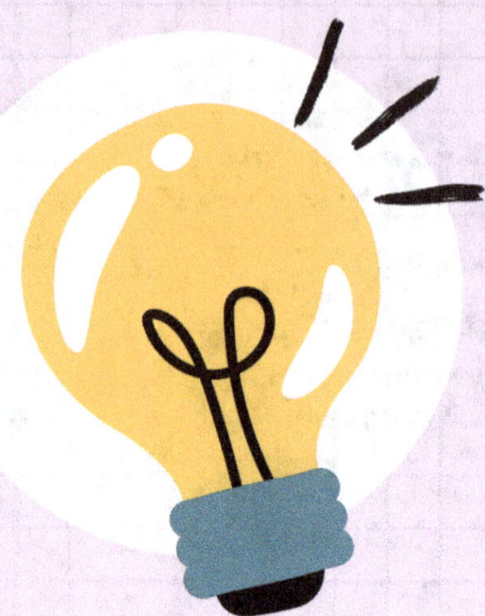

ANALYSIS

Lorem ipsum dolor sit amet, consectetur adipiscing elit. Suspendisse in mi sed velit lacinia vulputate. Vestibulum dignissim mollis ipsum sed pellentesque.

1

2

OBJECTIVES

Lorem ipsum dolor sit amet, consectetur adipiscing elit. Suspendisse in mi sed velit lacinia vulputate. Vestibulum dignissim mollis ipsum sed pellentesque.

STRATEGY

Lorem ipsum dolor sit amet, consectetur adipiscing elit. Suspendisse in mi sed velit lacinia vulputate. Vestibulum dignissim mollis ipsum sed pellentesque.

3

4

ACTION

Lorem ipsum dolor sit amet, consectetur adipiscing elit. Suspendisse in mi sed velit lacinia vulputate. Vestibulum dignissim mollis ipsum sed pellentesque.

REVISION

Lorem ipsum dolor sit amet, consectetur adipiscing elit. Suspendisse in mi sed velit lacinia vulputate. Vestibulum dignissim mollis ipsum sed pellentesque.

5

6

SOLUTION

Lorem ipsum dolor sit amet, consectetur adipiscing elit. Suspendisse in mi sed velit lacinia vulputate. Vestibulum dignissim mollis ipsum sed pellentesque.

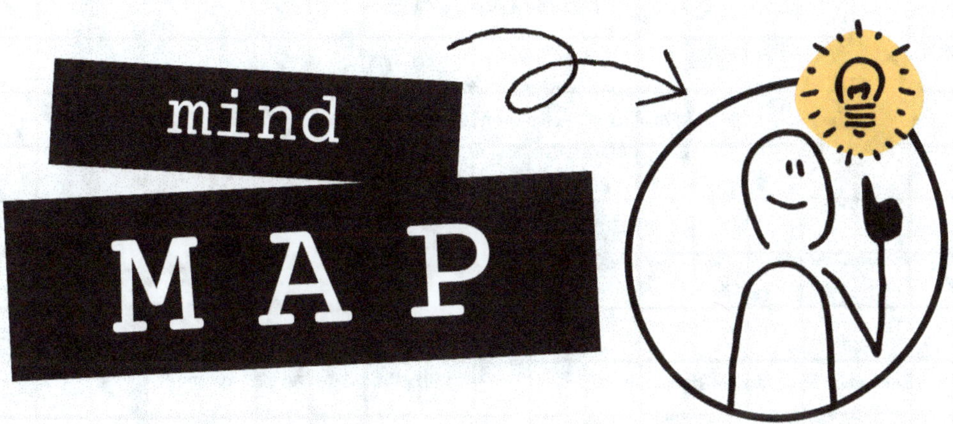

mind
MAP

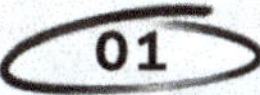

01

Analysis

Lorem ipsum dolor sit amet, consectetur adipiscing elit. Suspendisse in mi sed velit lacinia vulputate. Vestibulum dignissim mollis ipsum sed pellentesque.

02

Objectives

Lorem ipsum dolor sit amet, consectetur adipiscing elit. Suspendisse in mi sed velit lacinia vulputate. Vestibulum dignissim mollis ipsum sed pellentesque.

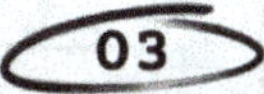

03

Strategy

Lorem ipsum dolor sit amet, consectetur adipiscing elit. Suspendisse in mi sed velit lacinia vulputate. Vestibulum dignissim mollis ipsum sed pellentesque.

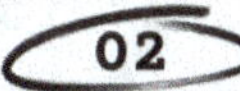

04

Action

Lorem ipsum dolor sit amet, consectetur adipiscing elit. Suspendisse in mi sed velit lacinia vulputate. Vestibulum dignissim mollis ipsum sed pellentesque.

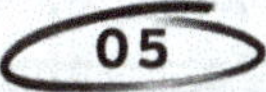

05

Revision

Lorem ipsum dolor sit amet, consectetur adipiscing elit. Suspendisse in mi sed velit lacinia vulputate. Vestibulum dignissim mollis ipsum sed pellentesque.

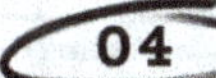

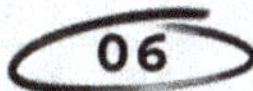

06

Solution

Lorem ipsum dolor sit amet, consectetur adipiscing elit. Suspendisse in mi sed velit lacinia vulputate. Vestibulum dignissim mollis ipsum sed pellentesque.

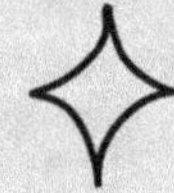

ORIGINAL IDEA

Lorem ipsum dolor sit amet consectetur adipiscing elit, euismod potenti cras pellentesque imperdiet luctus ridiculus, dis dapibus nunc porttitor eros hendrerit.

FRESH IDEA

Lorem ipsum dolor sit amet consectetur adipiscing elit, euismod potenti cras pellentesque imperdiet luctus ridiculus, dis dapibus nunc porttitor eros hendrerit.

SIMPLE IDEA

Lorem ipsum dolor sit amet consectetur adipiscing elit, euismod potenti cras pellentesque imperdiet luctus ridiculus, dis dapibus nunc porttitor eros hendrerit.

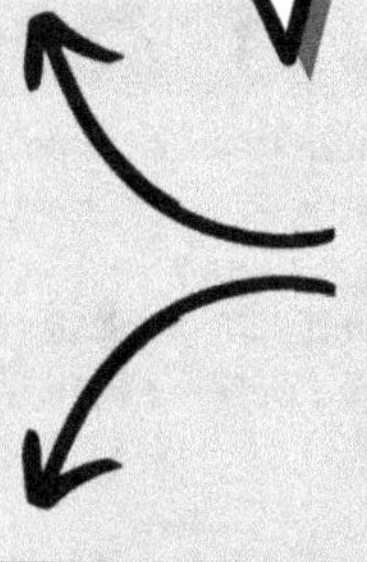
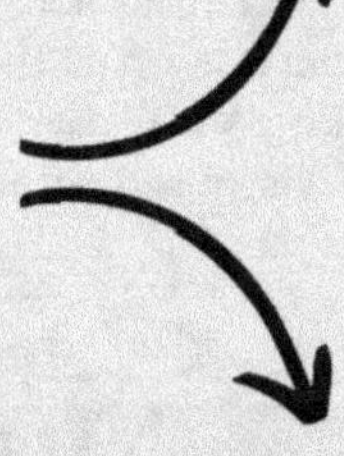

MIND MAP

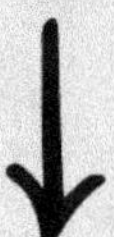

CLEVER IDEA

Lorem ipsum dolor sit amet consectetur adipiscing elit, euismod potenti cras pellentesque imperdiet luctus ridiculus, dis dapibus nunc porttitor eros hendrerit.

CREATIVE IDEA

Lorem ipsum dolor sit amet consectetur adipiscing elit, euismod potenti cras pellentesque imperdiet luctus ridiculus, dis dapibus nunc porttitor eros hendrerit.

UNIQUE IDEA

Lorem ipsum dolor sit amet consectetur adipiscing elit, euismod potenti cras pellentesque imperdiet luctus ridiculus, dis dapibus nunc porttitor eros hendrerit.

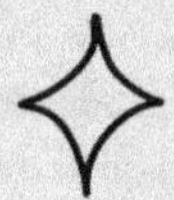
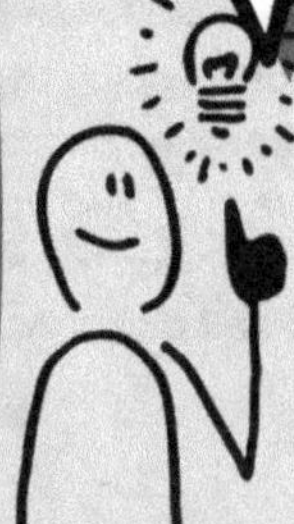

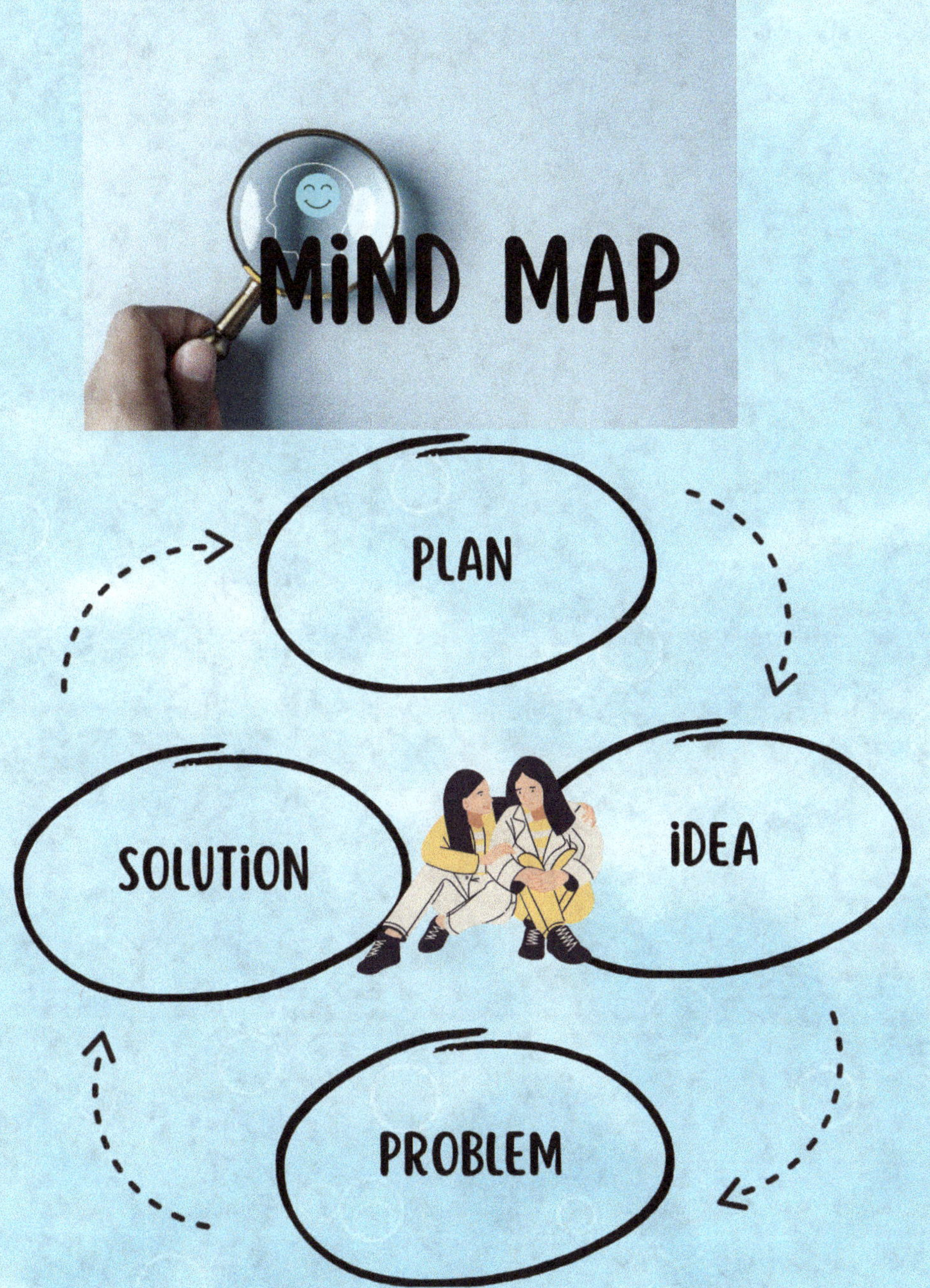

MIND MAP
PLAN
SOLUTION
IDEA
PROBLEM

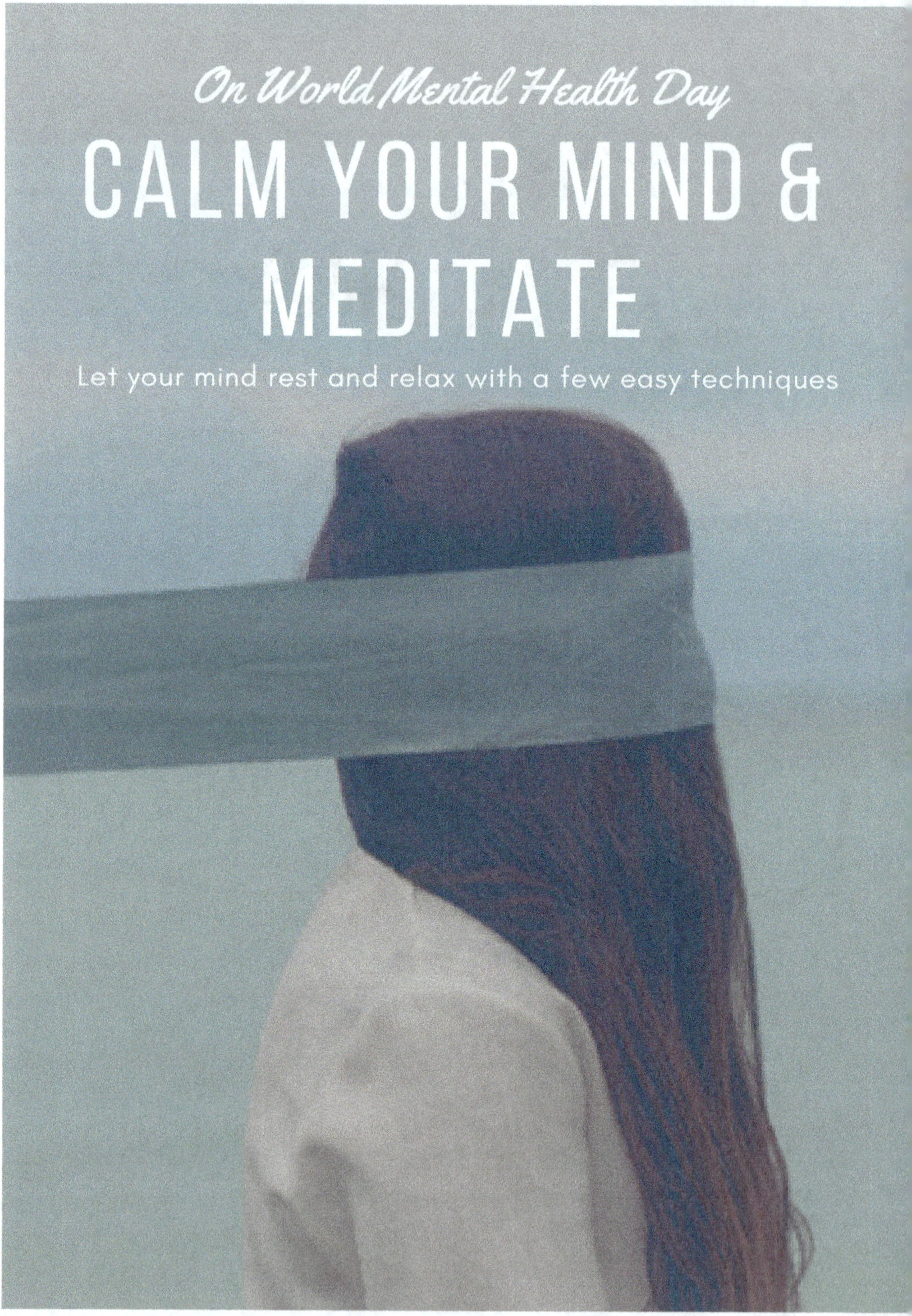

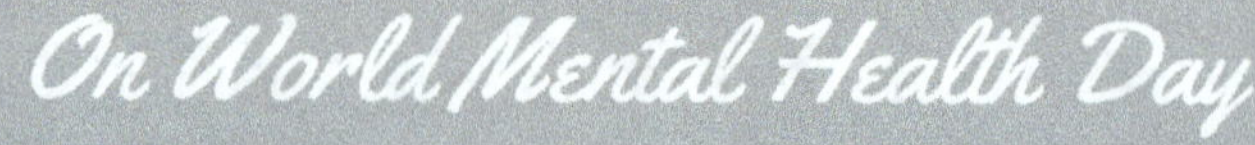

On World Mental Health Day
CALM YOUR MIND &
MEDITATE
Let your mind rest and relax with a few easy techniques

ALL ABOUT MENTAL HEALTH

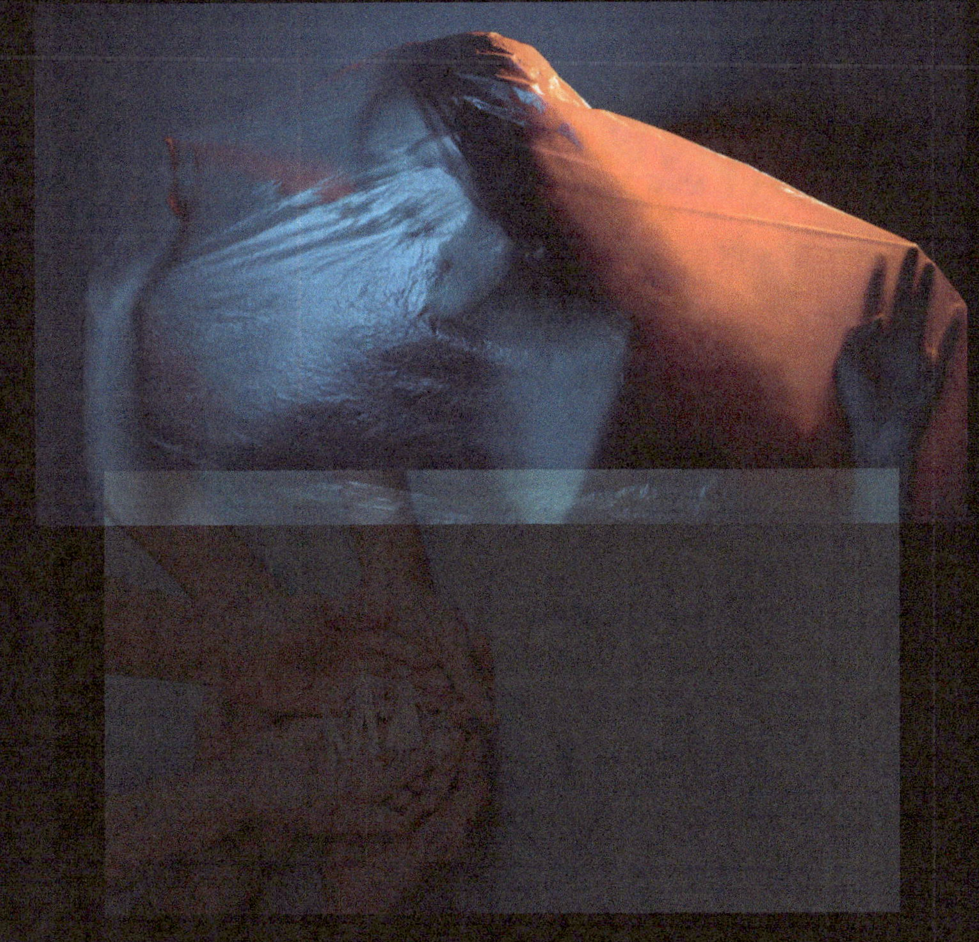

Talk
with Affirmations

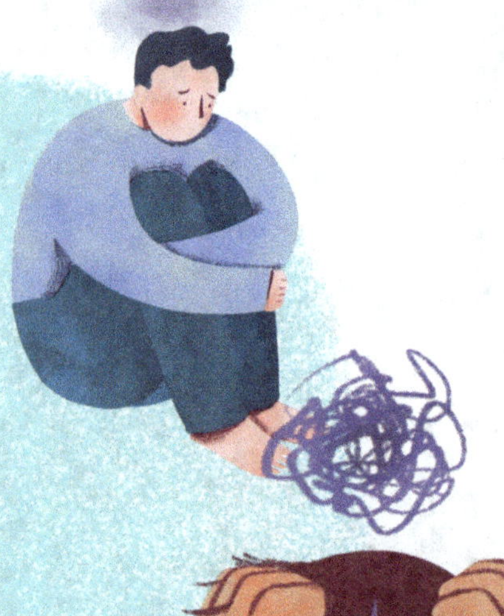

Create Positive Affirmations

Create positive affirmations that directly challenge those negative thoughts.

Identify Negative Self-Talk

Awareness is the first step in making a change.

Repeat and Internalize Affirmations

Repetition helps to reinforce positive beliefs and rewire your thought patterns over time.

Self Love & Mental Health

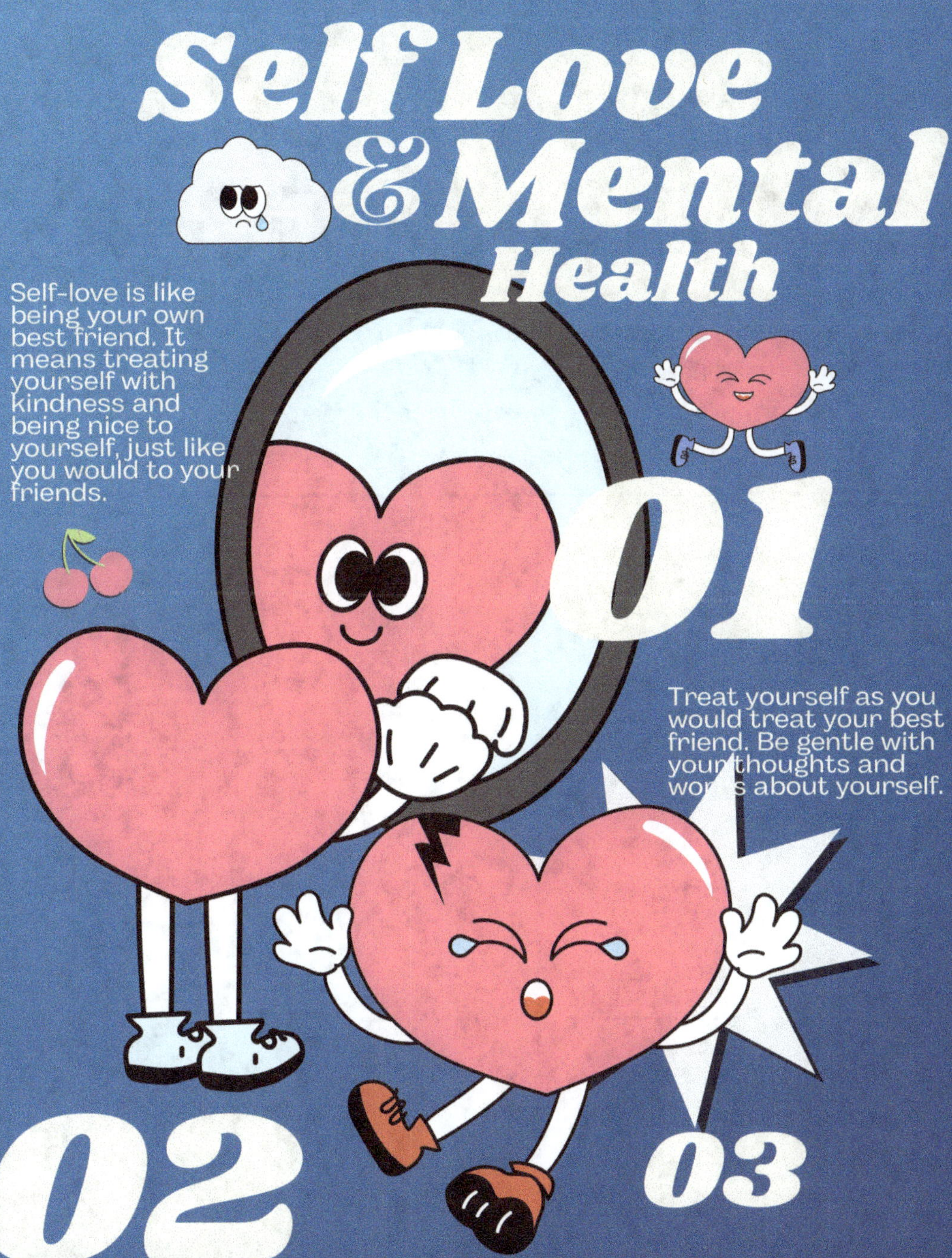

Self-love is like being your own best friend. It means treating yourself with kindness and being nice to yourself, just like you would to your friends.

01

Treat yourself as you would treat your best friend. Be gentle with your thoughts and words about yourself.

02

Say nice things to yourself, like "I am strong" or "I am capable." It's like giving yourself a pep talk.

03

Getting enough sleep is like recharging your brain. It helps you think clearly and feel less stressed.

Symptoms of Depression

Depression is a serious mental health condition that affects people from all walks of life. If you have symptoms, please seek help as there are many treatment options available.

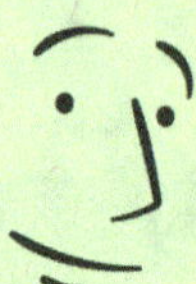

Insert first symptom

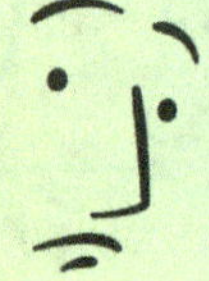

Insert second symptom

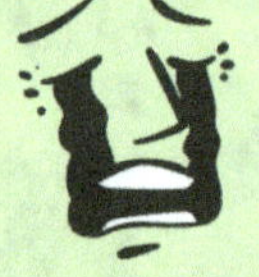

Insert third symptom

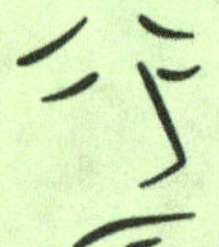

Insert fourth symptom

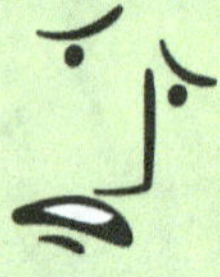

Insert fifth symptom

Insert sixth symptom

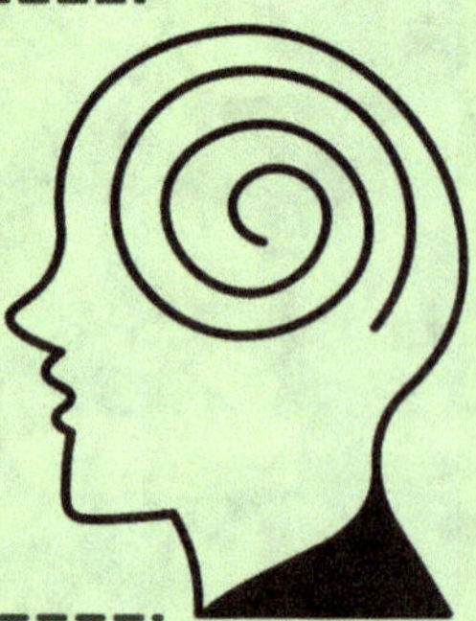

6 Effective Ways
TO STUDY BETTER

3 VARIED STUDY METHODS

Utilize different study techniques, such as reading, note-taking, flashcards, and practice questions, to reinforce learning through various approaches.

2 ACTIVE LEARNING

Engage actively with the material through methods like summarizing information, teaching concepts to others, and participating in discussions.

4 HEALTHY ENVIRONMENT

Choose a comfortable and well-lit study environment, minimizing distractions to enhance focus and concentration.

1 EFFECTIVE PLANNING

Create a study schedule that breaks down your tasks into manageable sessions, ensuring a balance between subjects and topics

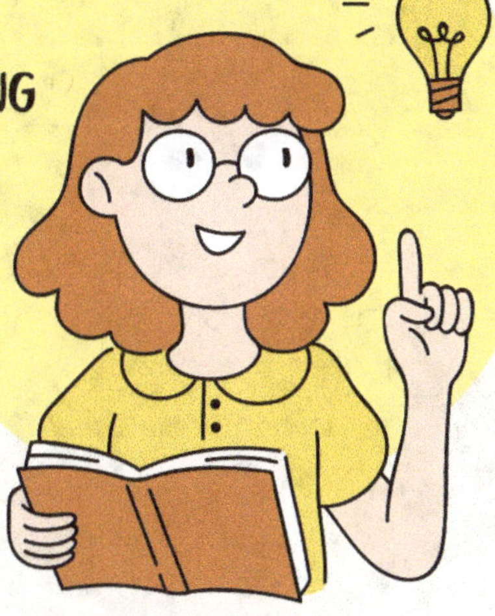

5 REGULAR BREAKS

Take short breaks during study sessions to prevent mental fatigue and maintain overall productivity.

6 SELF-ASSESSMENT

Regularly evaluate your understanding of the material through self-assessment tools, quizzes, or practice exams to identify areas that need further review.

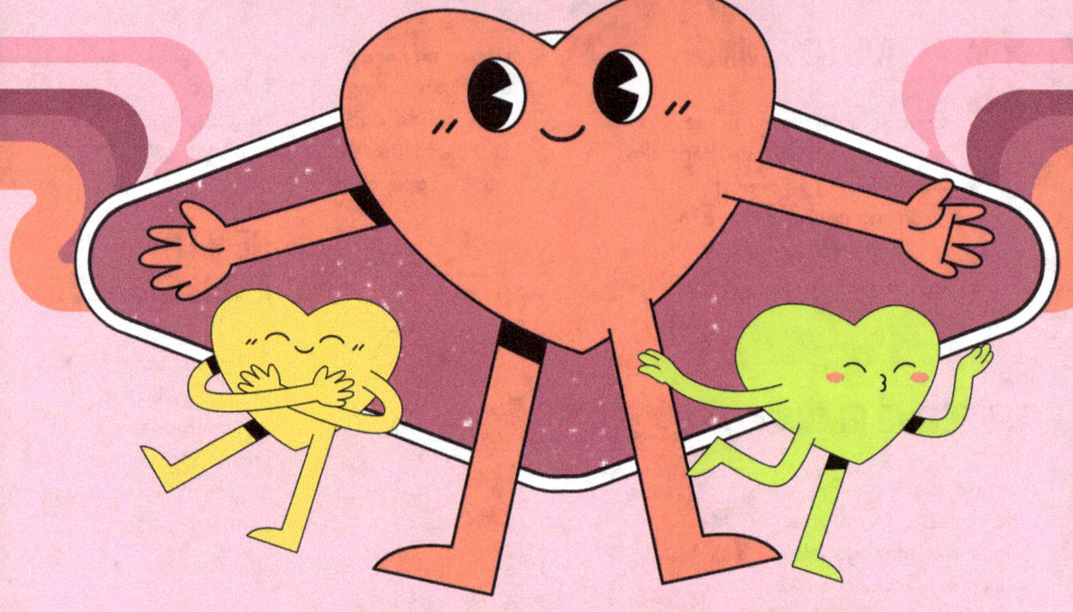

COMPARISON AND ENVY

It can make you unhappy because you're focusing on what you lack instead of appreciating what you have.

DWELLING ON THE PAST

It can make you unhappy because it keeps you stuck in those negative moments instead of moving forward.

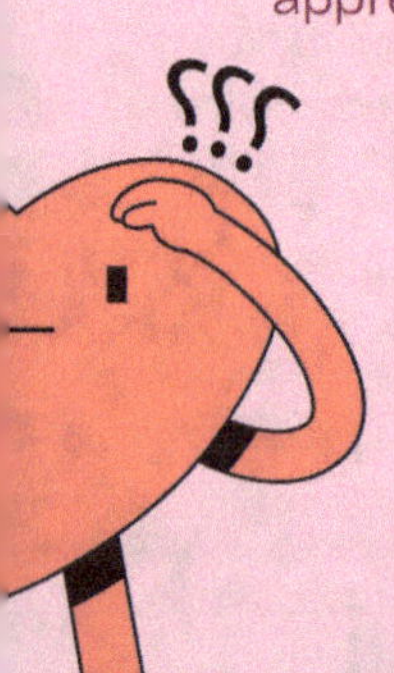

NEGATIVE SELF-TALK

It can make you unhappy because it lowers your self-esteem and makes you feel bad about yourself.

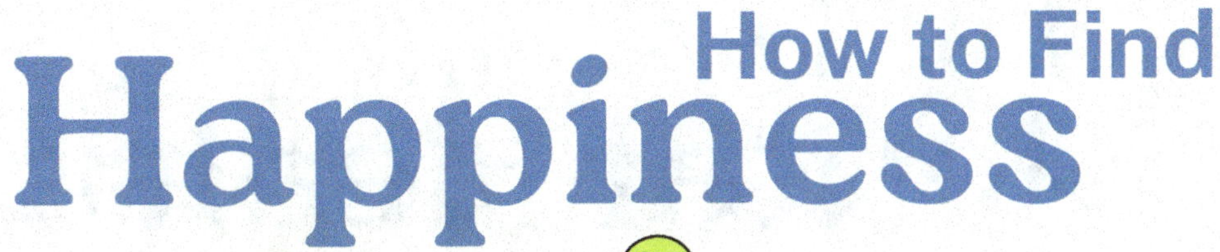

How to Find Happiness

Learn and Grow

Always try new things or learn something new. It feels good to achieve something and learn from it. That feeling can make you happy.

Stop Chasing Happiness

Sometimes, if you try too hard to be happy, it's harder to find. Instead, focus on doing things that make you feel good inside.

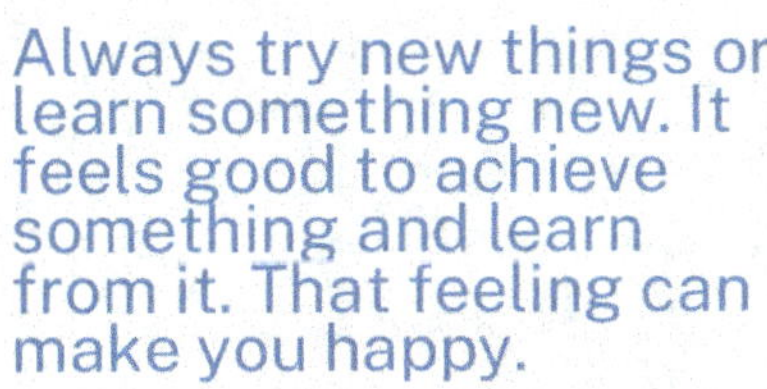

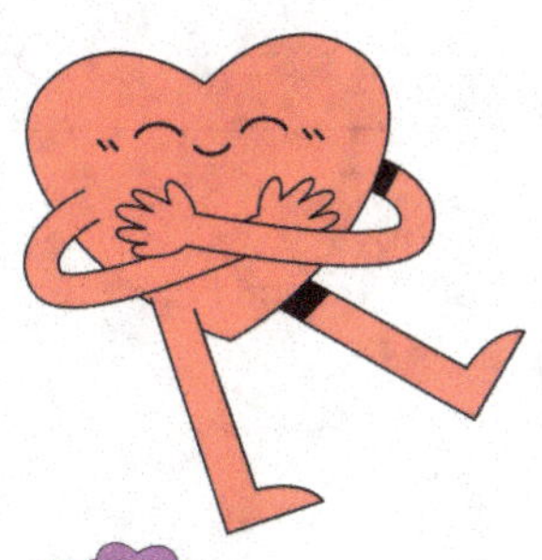

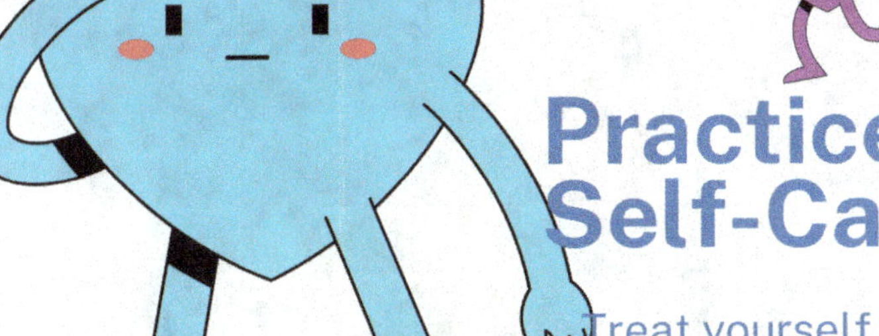

Practice Self-Care

Treat yourself well. Do things that make you feel relaxed or happy, like taking a walk, reading a book, or spending time with friends.

Self-Love and Mental Health

Self-love is an ongoing practice and involves nurturing a positive relationship with yourself. It's important to prioritize self-care, seek support when needed, and cultivate self-compassion.

Self-love entails establishing healthy boundaries, confidently saying 'no' when necessary, and giving precedence to one's needs and well-being, all without feeling guilty.

Self-love also encompasses self-compassion, wherein individuals treat themselves with kindness and understanding during trying times or when confronted with setbacks.

Engaging in self-love practices can enhance mental health by bolstering self-esteem, self-confidence, and resilience in the face of challenges.

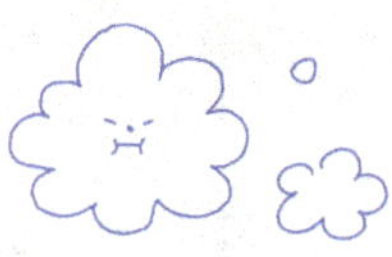

Self-love is the act of nurturing and valuing oneself. It encompasses embracing both strengths and weaknesses while making self-care a priority.

By prioritising self-love, you can enhance your mental well-being and lead a healthier, more fulfilling life.

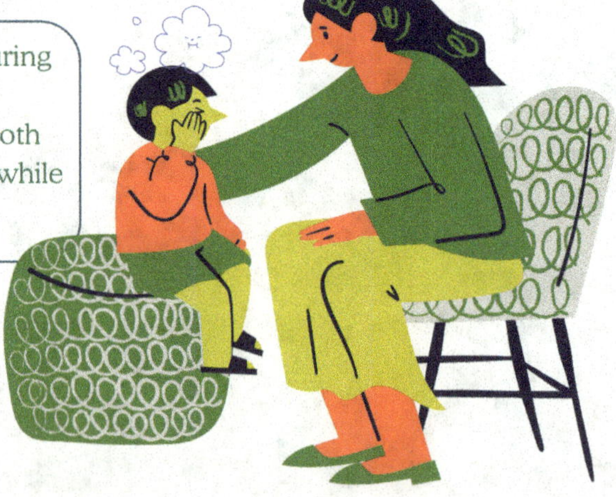

BUILDING RESILIENCE AND MENTAL STRENGTH

01

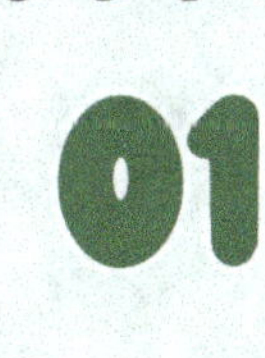
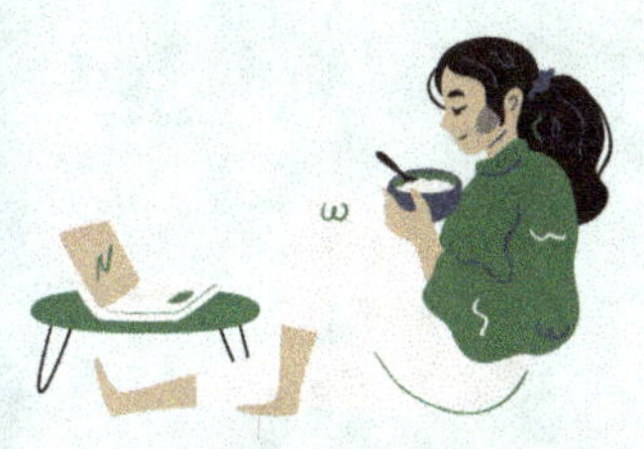

Resilience is the ability to adapt, bounce back, and recover from adversity, trauma, or significant life challenges

02

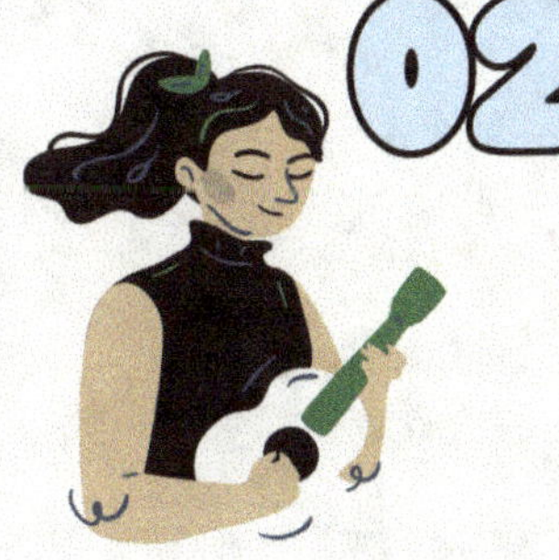

Building resilience involves developing a positive mindset, focusing on strengths, and cultivating optimism even in challenging situations.

Resilience can be nurtured through self-care practices. You can exercise, get enough sleep, healthy eating, and engage in activities that bring joy and relaxation.

03

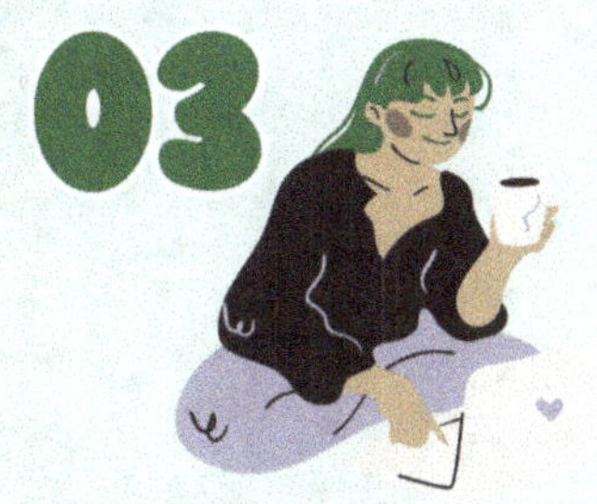

04

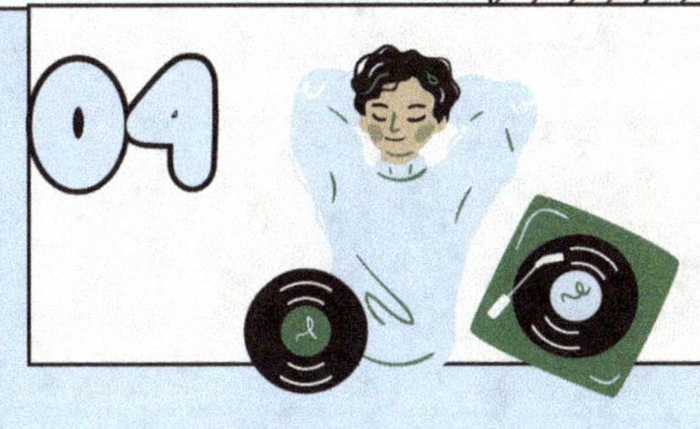

Building a strong support system with friends, family, or support groups can enhance resilience by providing emotional support, understanding, and encouragement.

THINGS TO
Remember

It's okay to
take
a break.

You're free
to be
different.

Anything
worth having
takes time.

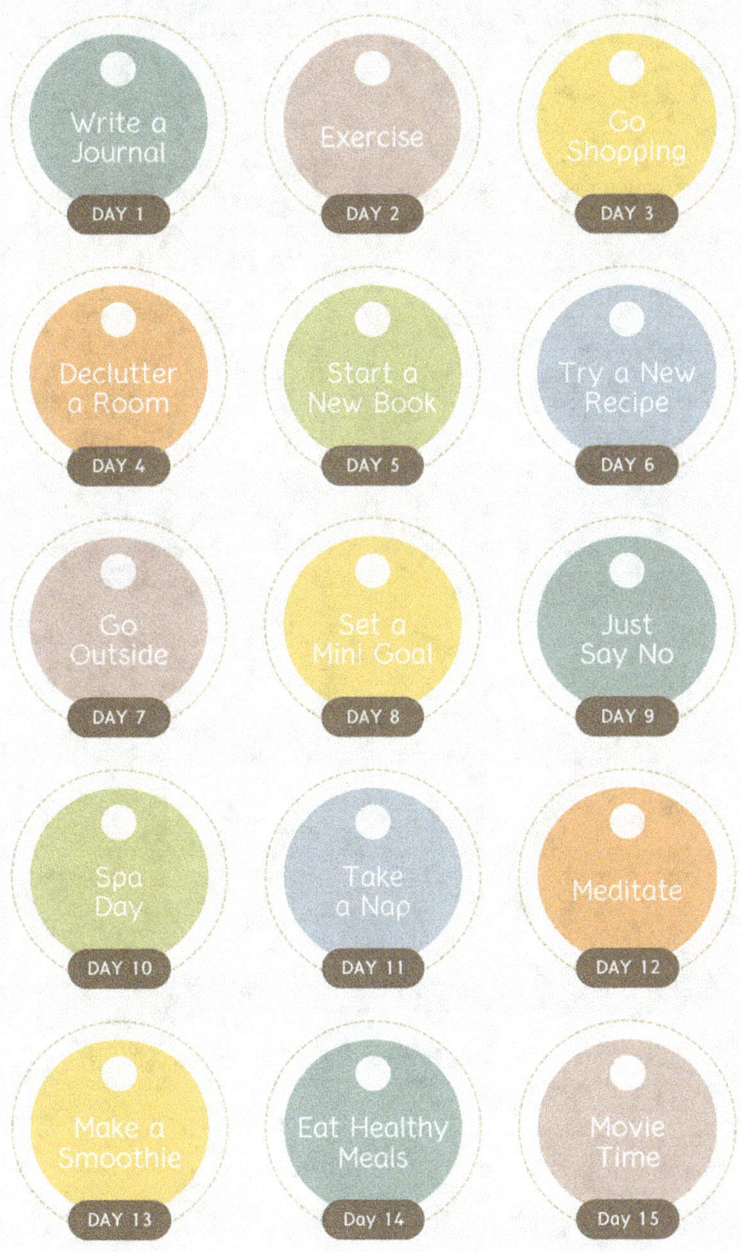

15 DAY
Self-Care Challenge
Write a Journal
DAY 1
Exercise
DAY 2
Go Shopping
DAY 3
Declutter a Room
DAY 4
Start a New Book
DAY 5
Try a New Recipe
DAY 6
Go Outside
DAY 7
Set a Mini Goal
DAY 8
Just Say No
DAY 9
Spa Day
DAY 10
Take a Nap
DAY 11
Meditate
DAY 12
Make a Smoothie
DAY 13
Eat Healthy Meals
Day 14
Movie Time
Day 15

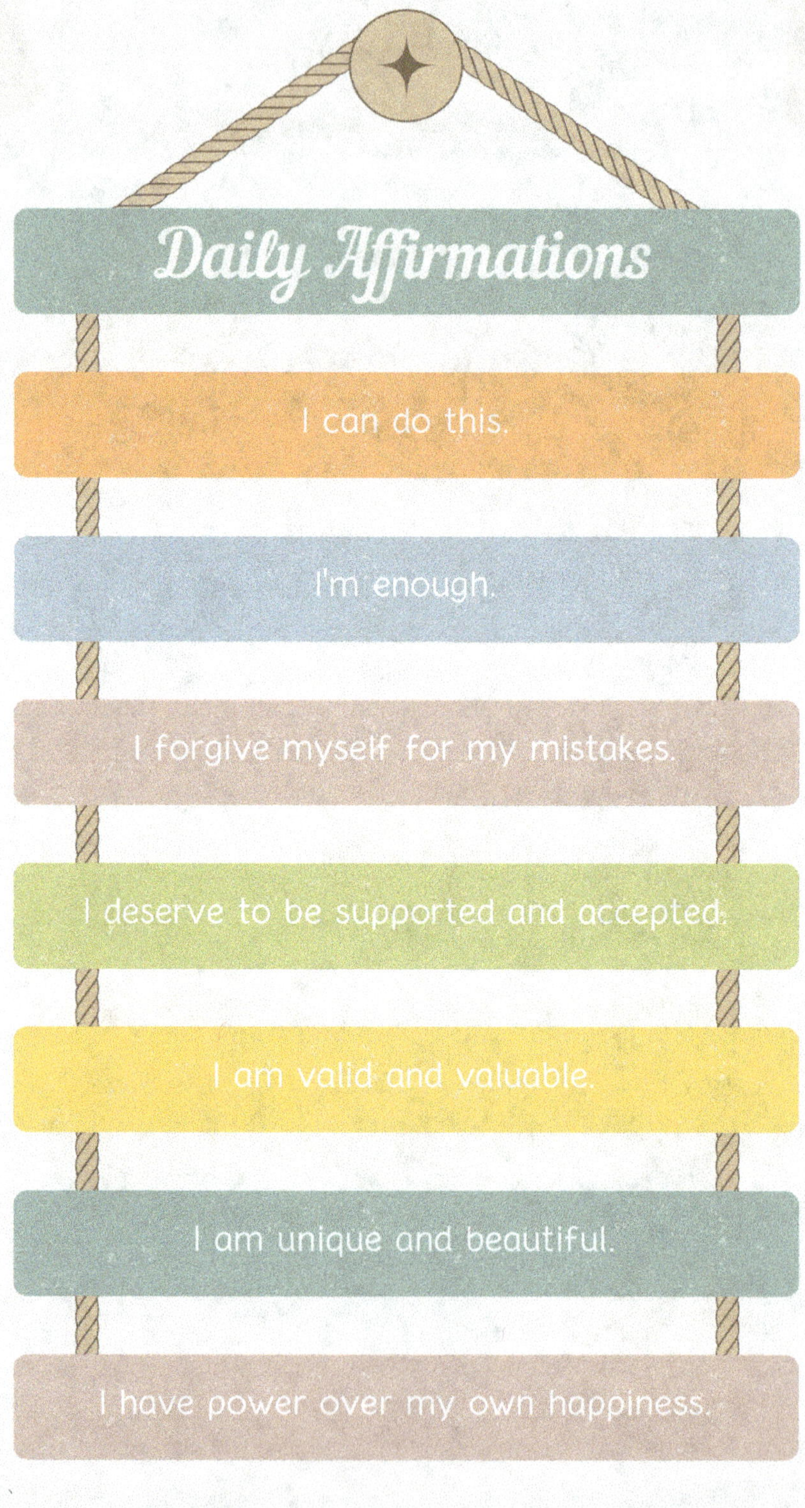

Daily Affirmations
I can do this.
I'm enough.
I forgive myself for my mistakes.
I deserve to be supported and accepted.
I am valid and valuable.
I am unique and beautiful.
I have power over my own happiness.

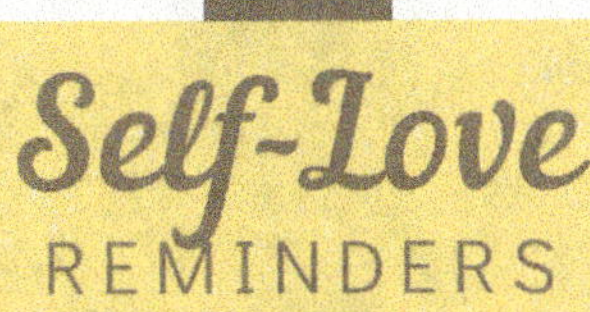

Self-Love
REMINDERS

01 " It's okay to take a break.

" You're free to be different. 02

03 " Anything worth having takes time.

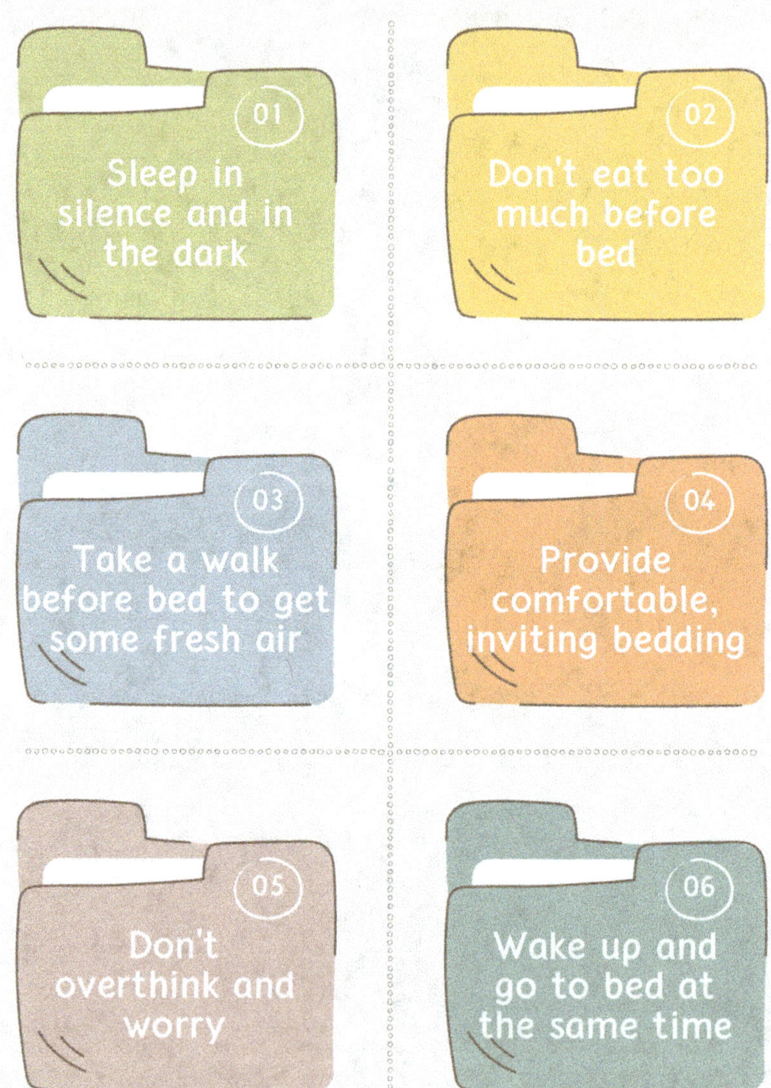

Sleeping Tips
FOR A HEALTHY LIFE
01
Sleep in silence and in the dark
02
Don't eat too much before bed
03
Take a walk before bed to get some fresh air
04
Provide comfortable, inviting bedding
05
Don't overthink and worry
06
Wake up and go to bed at the same time

How to Get *Healthy Skin*

1. Protect yourself from the sun

2. Treat your skin gently

3. Eat a healthy diet

4. Keep stress in check

5. Keep moisture in the skin

5 TIPS FOR
EXAM PREPARATION

Plan a study timetable

Prepare your study area

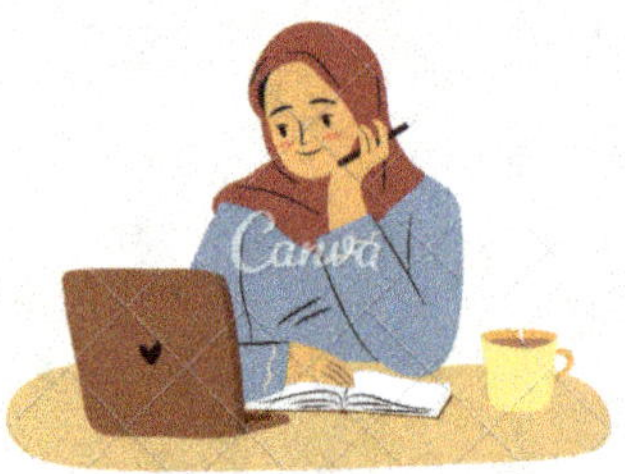

Keep healthy eat, sleep and move

Minimise distractions and overcome procrastination

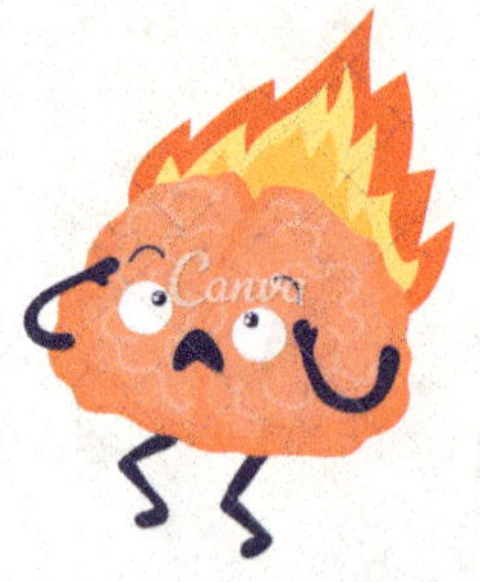

Take breaks for your wellbeing

Self Love & Mental Health

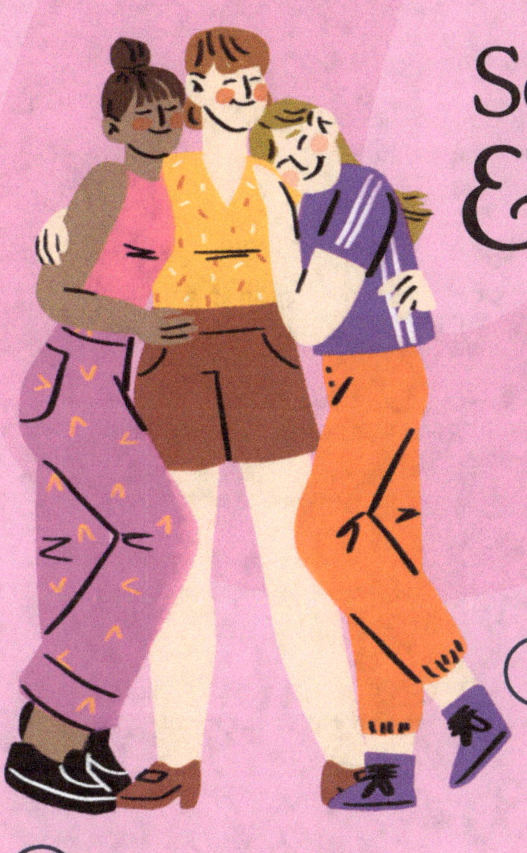

1

Self-love is a practice of nurturing and valuing oneself. It includes accepting both strengths and weaknesses and prioritizing self-care.

2

Practicing self-love can improve mental health by boosting self-esteem, self-confidence, and resilience in the face of challenges.

3

Self-love involves setting healthy boundaries, saying no when necessary, and prioritizing one's own needs and well-being without guilt.

4

Self-love includes practicing self-compassion and treating oneself with kindness and understanding during difficult times or when facing setbacks.

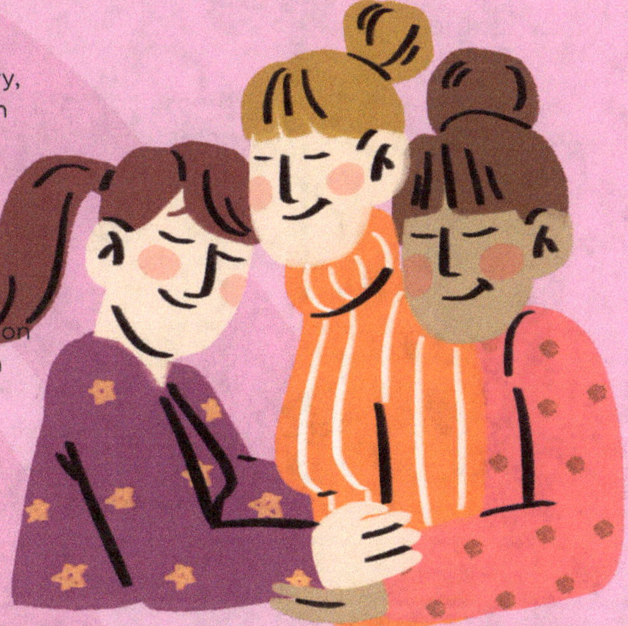

My Safety Plan

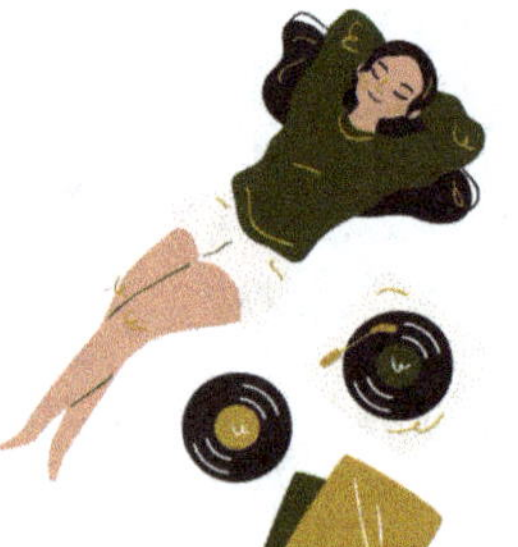

Remember:
Help is always available.

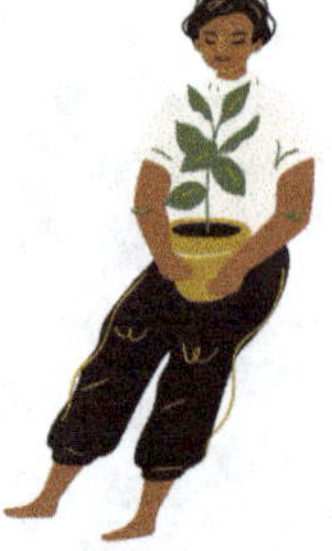

1 My warning signs are:

*These can be thoughts, feelings or behaviors that indicate you are at risk.

2 My effective coping strategies are:

*These are things you can do to help lift your mood, like meditation or exercise.

3 People I can reach out to for distraction:

4 People I can reach out to for help:

5 Steps I can take to make my environment safer. Please list:

6 In the event of a crisis:

Call Emergency Contact #1:

Call Crisis Hotline:

Call Emergency Services:

WHAT DO YOU KNOW ABOUT ANXIETY?

56% of people in the U.S. think we are more anxious today than 5 years ago.

Anxiety is a common emotion experienced by many people at some point in their lives. It is a feeling of worry, nervousness, or unease about something with an uncertain outcome. Anxiety can manifest in physical symptoms such as increased heart rate, sweating, trembling, and difficulty breathing. It's important to remember that experiencing anxiety is a normal part of being human, but when it becomes overwhelming and starts interfering with daily life, it may be a sign of an anxiety disorder that could benefit from professional help. There are various ways to manage anxiety, including therapy, medication, relaxation techniques, exercise, and mindfulness practices. It's essential to prioritize self-care and seek support from loved ones or mental health professionals if needed. Remember, you are not alone in your struggles, and there are resources available to help you navigate through your anxiety.

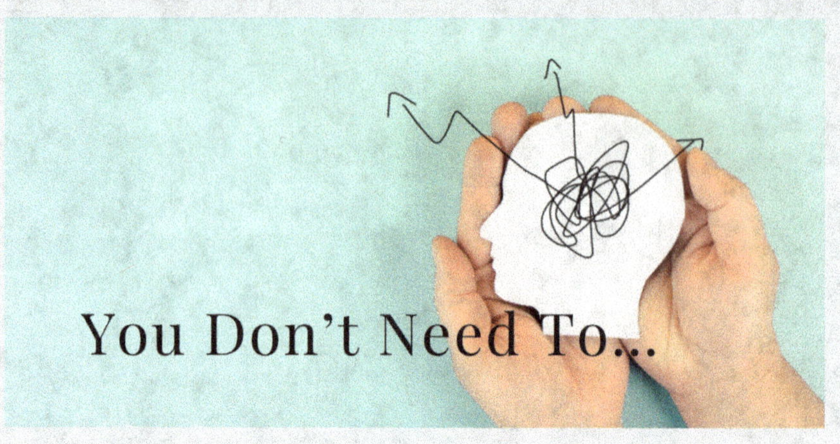

STAY IN THE PAST

KEEP EVERYONE HAPPY

PUSH YOURSELF BEYOND THE LIMIT

OVERTHINK EVERYTHING

IGNORE YOUR EMOTIONS

SACRIFICE YOUR HEALTH

#SelfCare

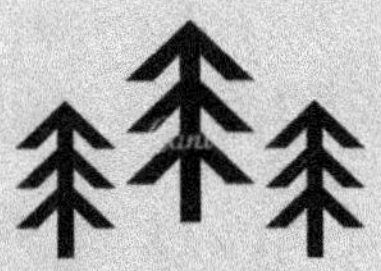

SEE & EXPLORE

THE
WORLD
IS YOUR
OYSTER.

the perfect time is now

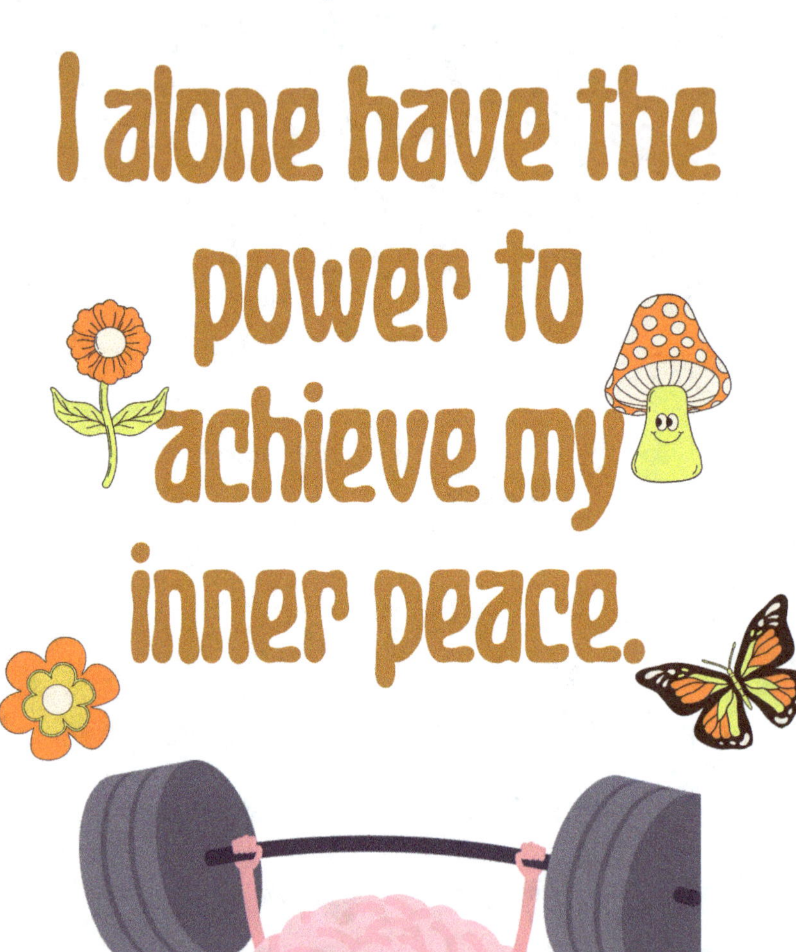

I alone have the power to achieve my inner peace.

YOU HAVE THE POWER TO PROTECT YOUR PEACE

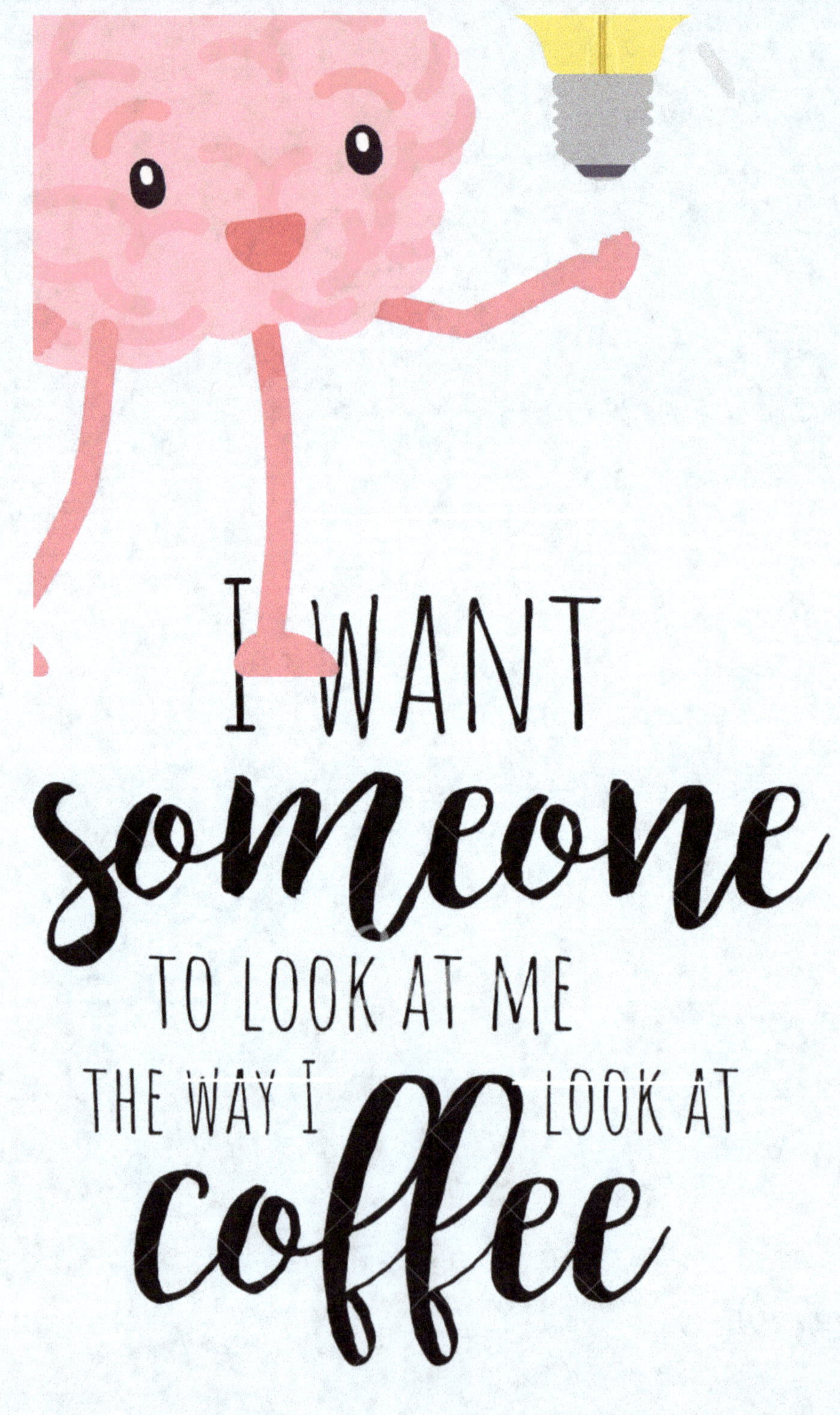
I WANT
someone
TO LOOK AT ME
THE WAY I LOOK AT
coffee

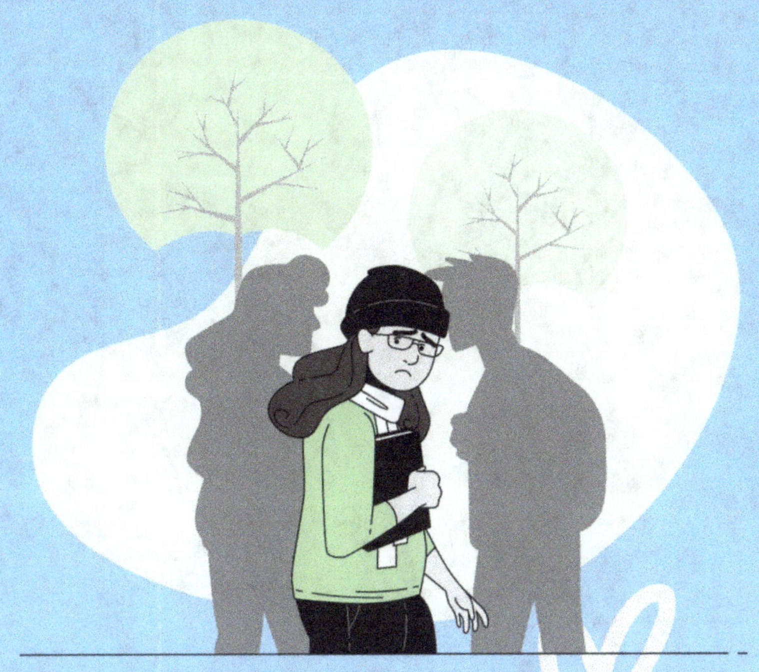

YOU ARE
enough.

Anything
WORTH
HAVING
Takes
TIME

KEEP IT SIMPLE

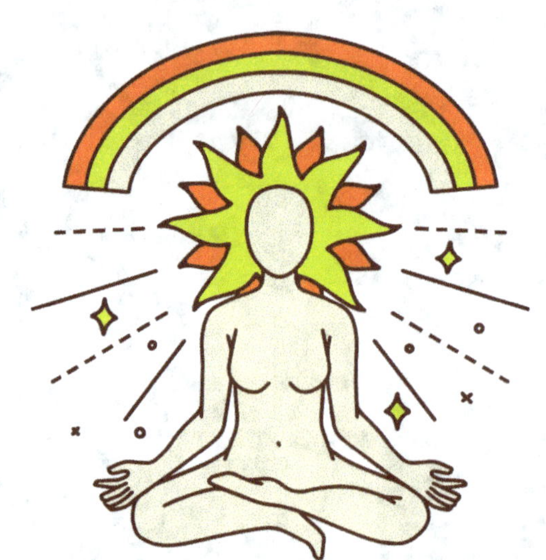
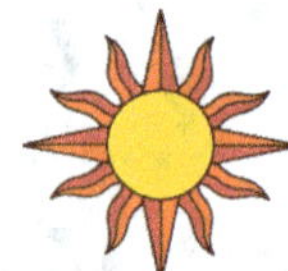
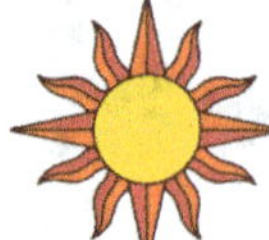

I AM TRUSTING IN THE TIMING OF THE UNIVERSE.

YOU DON'T HAVE TO BE POSITIVE TO THINK

POSITIVE

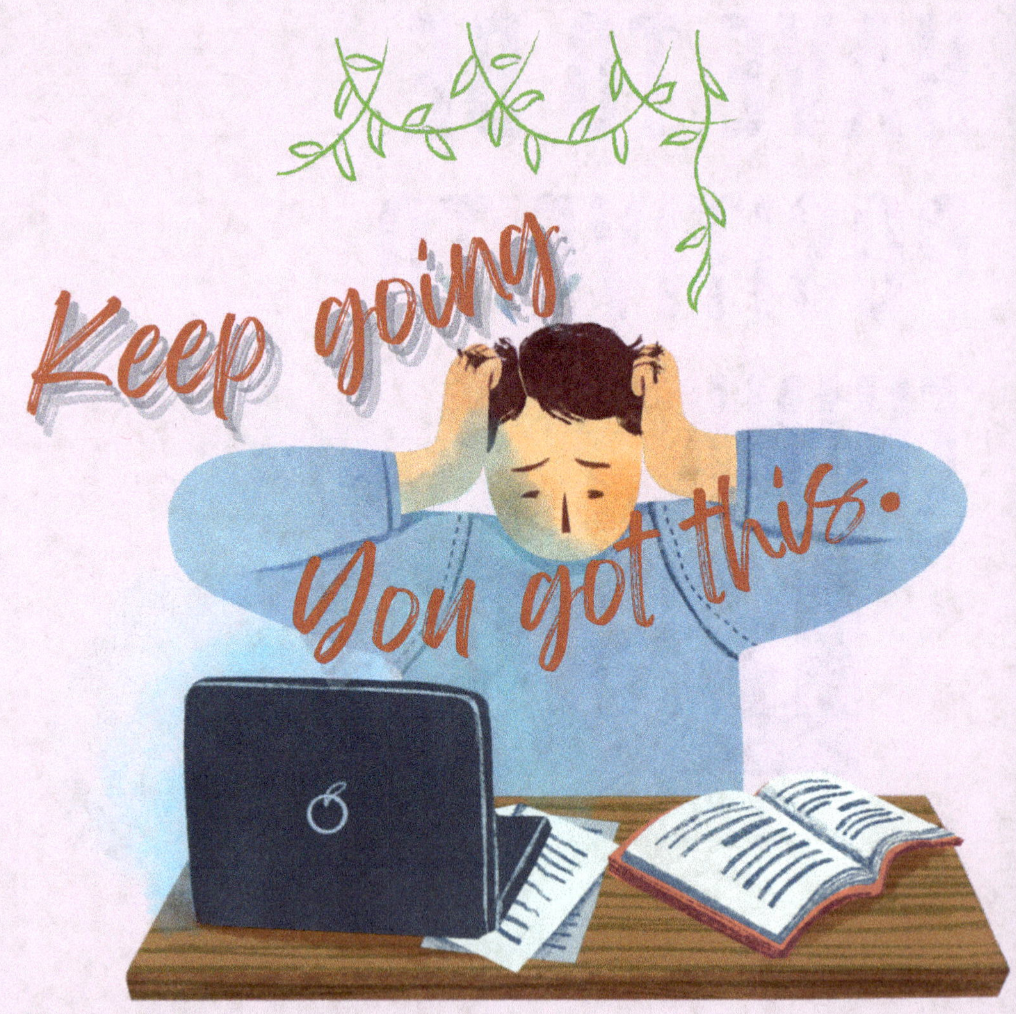
Keep going
You got this.

Supporting Others:
- How to be an ally
- Providing emotional support
- Encouraging professional help-seeking
Conclusion:
- Emphasizing that mental health is a journey
- Encouraging hope and perseverance
- Reminding readers that they are not alone

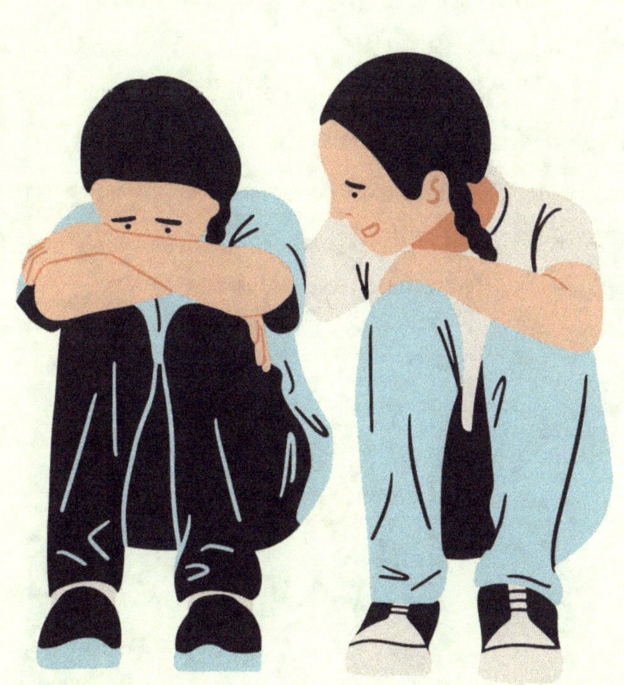

CONCLUSION

Self-care is an integral part of maintaining your overall well-being. It involves taking care of your physical, mental, and emotional needs and finding ways to relax and unwind. There are many different self-care strategies that you can use, such as getting enough sleep, exercising regularly, practicing mindfulness, and engaging in activities that bring you joy. It's also essential to seek support, whether talking to a loved one, seeing a therapist, or joining a support group. By regularly incorporating self-care into your routine and seeking support when needed, you can help to maintain your overall well-being and feel more balanced and fulfilled.

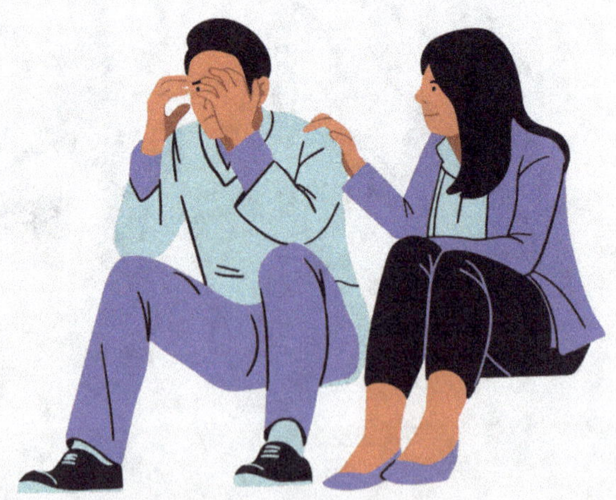